KING'S
Guide to TENS
for Health Professionals

A Health Professionals' Guide
to Transcutaneous Electrical Nerve Stimulation
for the Treatment of Pain

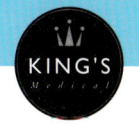

Alan King

Grad Dip Phys. MCSP. SRP.

By the same author:

King's Guide to TENS
A Users Guide to Transcutaneous Electrical Nerve Stimulation
ISBN 0-9535623-0-1

King's Pocket Book of Acupuncture Points For TENS and Other Methods of Stimulation
A Health Professional's Guide
ISBN 0-9535623-1-X

First Edition
Published by Kings Medical
ISBN 0-9535623-2-8

© Alan King, 1999
Registered at Stationer's Hall
All Rights Reserved

No part of this publication may be reproduced, stored in a retrieval system or transmitted in any form, or by any means, without the prior permission, in writing, of the publisher; nor be otherwise circulated in any form of binding or cover other than that in which it is published and without a similar condition, including this condition, being imposed on the subsequent purchaser.

Every care has been taken throughout this book to ensure the accuracy of information but the publisher cannot accept responsibility for any errors that may appear.

Designed and Illustrated by ***David J. Elliott***

Contents

Page	
7	Introduction.
8	The Genesis of TENS
9	TENS today
10-11	Why use TENS?
12	An Overview of TENS
12	Contra-indications and Cautions
13-14	Pain, a Definition and Types of Pain
14-16	Pain Pathways and the Associated Nerves
17-19	Peripheral Nerves and Functions
20	Nerves of the Central Nervous System
21	TENS and the Neuromodulation of Pain
22	The TENS Machine, its controls and output
	Setting the TENS for:
26-27	a) Pain Gating
28-30	b) Endorphin Production
	Other Variables:
30-32	a) Polarity
32-35	b) Electrode Positioning (finding vertebrae and dermatome maps)
36	c) Treatments - How long and how often?
37	The Pain Gate vs. Endorphin Production
38-39	Indications for Treatment
40-45	Notes, Assessment and Re-assessment
46	Anti-emisis
47	Side Effects
48	Choosing Equipment
48-49	a) The TENS Machine
49	b) Other Equipment
50-53	Information for Patients
54-55	Electrode Position Maps
56-57	References
58	Index

Introduction

In pain management TENS, if used correctly, does work!

Pulsed electrical stimulation via surface electrodes excites specific nerves which undergo temporal change, mediate changes at spinal cord level, and further, will stimulate changes in higher centres. These changes - in isolation or in combination - enhance pain management.

Transcutaneous Electrical Nerve Stimulation (TENS) is still a much under-used modality. Clinicians may avoid its use due to inadequacies in post-graduate training. Others, who have tried TENS without success, may push it to one side in favour of better known and regularly used alternatives.

Many patients who visited the pain clinic in which the author practised had previously tried TENS without significantly affecting their pain. Upon questioning, it was discovered that they had attempted to follow the supplier's pamphlet or had been poorly instructed in both the application and effects of TENS. They were understandably reluctant to re-try TENS. Perhaps these factors underline the need for an improved understanding of TENS. This text is aimed at those clinicians who wish to improve their pain management skills, and therefore the welfare of their patients, by adding TENS to the other modalities that they are familiar with. The group in mind encompasses G.P's, hospital doctors, physiotherapists, and nurses including those working in the community, all of whom may be involved in acute and chronic pain management.

Managing pain employing TENS is not a panacea for all ills. However, approaching the problem in a systamatic and structured manner, providing the necessary information and support, will give your patients the best opportunity to achieve significant pain management.

The Genesis of TENS

Electrical stimulation, in one form or another, has been carried out by humans since before the time of the Egyptian Empire. Sufferers of painful gout were stimulated with the electrical discharges of torpedo fish in an attempt to moderate their pain.

The practice of electrical stimulation continued up to the early 1960's without any real theories of how it worked until the publication of the gate control theory of pain by *Melzack & Wall (1)*. This theory suggested that stimulation of the large diameter afferent nerves modulate the information carried by the smaller afferent nerves. It is suggested that the modulation occurs within the dorsal horn (*Substantia Gelatinosa*) of the spinal cord. As the smaller nerve fibres are responsible for carrying information on pain, this in turn would reduce the volume of 'painful traffic' reaching the higher centres and therefore the perception of pain.

TENS was originally developed as a device to test the probability of success of Dorsal Column Stimulation (DCS). DCS was a technique of electrical stimulation which was used in an attempt to ameliorate chronic pain that had not responded to more conventional measures. It involved the implantation of electrodes in the spinal cord which were then electrically stimulated via wires from a signal generator. This technique involved a surgical procedure - with its inherent risks.

TENS, which may be described as a pulse signal generator, was applied using only surface applied electrodes. It was found that TENS in isolation produced pain management without the need to go on to DCS and implantation. *Eriksson et al (2)* suggested that TENS should be tried as a therapy before considering implantable devices or destructive surgery.

TENS has continued to be developed as a further tool for pain management.

TENS Today

TENS today is a portable battery driven device which produces a variable pulsed electrical signal which is carried via leads to electrodes placed on the skin. The activity in these will in turn stimulate the underlying nerves.

Careful positioning of the electrodes over appropriate nerve bundles ensures stimulation of the targeted segment. Adjustment of the machine's controls allows the clinician to select the physiological mechanism by which pain management may be achieved.

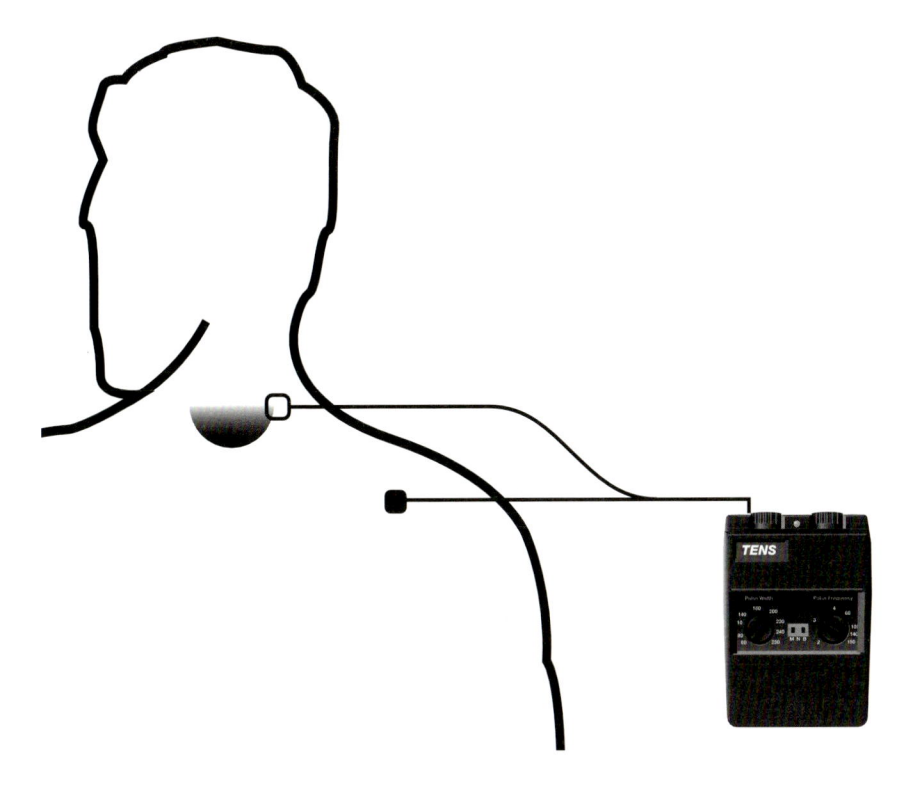

Why Use TENS?

EMPOWERING THE PATIENT
Possibly one of the most important reasons to employ TENS is that it puts pain management in the hands of the patient.

PATIENT-BASED
Following the initial visit and assessment, most patients can achieve competent TENS use after a period of five reviews spaced at intervals of one week. They may then decide when and for how long they wish to use TENS. Any further reviews that may be necessary can be spaced up to 3 or 6 months apart. This has a cost saving implication. (Short-term loan machines should be made available to each patient.)

SIDE EFFECTS
Other than allergies to the electrode gels and adhesives (which can usually be resolved), there are very few side effects.

LOW INITIAL COST
After a successful trial period, the patient may be encouraged to purchase their own machine. This may cost as little as £35.00.

LOW COST of CONSUMABLES
Some of the newly introduced reusable electrodes have an extended life of several months. With care, the lead wires may last longer than six months. Batteries will usually continue to be serviceable for up to eight weeks, depending upon levels of use.

NON-INVASIVE
Nobody *enjoys* injections. Patients are often reluctant to continue taking medication for extended periods. The effects of long term NSAI (non-steroidal anti-inflammatories) use are well known.

MOBILITY

The psychological effects of improved mobility are augmented with the physiological effects of normal movement which may further enhance afferent flow in the large diameter nerves also helping to maintain pain management.

'Selling' the Idea of TENS to the Patient

TENS is not a panacea for all pains, nor is it a cure. If properly applied, TENS will reduce pain by a significant amount in a significant number of people, allowing them to achieve a much improved quality of life. It is important that this is stressed before trials commence for, if the patient's expectation is that of a cure, anything less may be considered as failure. The practitioner may also consider these points.

About This Book

The clinician can only satisfy the needs of the patient if they themselves have a comprehensive understanding of the mechanisms of TENS. This understanding must encompass the effects of peripheral stimulation on both the peripheral and central nervous system.

This book is intended to provide the clinician with the basic information necessary to employ TENS in a structured manner in both clinical and domestic settings.
A comprehensive text on TENS has already been produced by *Walsh (3)*. This book is essential reading for those involved in pain clinics and/or research and a valuable reference book for all clinicians using TENS.

TENS Overview

The TENS machine itself could be described as a Pulse Signal Generator. The output of the machine is variable in amplitude and some variations in signal. The clinician/patient may select whether pain control is mediated by **pain-gating / dynorphin production** or by the production of **endogenous opioids** by selecting specific stimulation parameters with adjustments made on the TENS machine. These are described in the section *Setting the TENS*.

The signal from the TENS machine is conducted in fine wires to the electrodes which are adherent to the skin. The pulsed current at the electrodes excites the underlying nerve bundles which in turn will convey action potentials both proximally and distally. The proximal propagation of action potentials will arrive at the spinal cord in the region of the posterior horn. This is where pain gating is postulated to occur mediated by a specific set of stimulation parameters.

A change in stimulation parameters, (detailed in a later section) is thought to cause excitation of a first and second order of neurone that will, in turn, excite higher centres in the brain itself. It is thought that it is this mechanism which causes the release of endogenous opioids. *Han (4).* The nerve bundles stimulated, and hence the individual nerves and spinal segments, will be dependent upon the electrode site chosen.

To achieve effective use of TENS, one must appreciate pain types, (acute and chronic) the nerve pathways in which pain and other sensation is conveyed from the peripheral to the central nervous system, and the physiological effects of peripheral stimulation on both the peripheral and central nervous systems.

The following sections describe pain, the peripheral nerves, the TENS machine, and the appropriate physiology. Each of these points will combine to provide a basic understanding of the mechanisms of TENS.

Contra-indications

a) One of the main contra-indications to TENS use is in the group of people who have a pacemaker fitted. There is a danger that the output from the TENS machine may interfere with pacemaker function.
b) Fragile or broken skin where the electrodes are to be placed.
c) The presence of a percutaneous central venous catheter.
d) When driving or operating machinery.

Cautions

i) There is a theoretical risk in the first trimester of pregnancy.
ii) Do not place electrodes over the carotid sinuses as this may cause a significant drop in blood pressure.
iii) In the early stages of TENS use, it is prudent to observe the skin for any signs of allergic reactions.

Pain

Pain is extremely difficult to define. However, many attempts have been made and the following is now the accepted definition:

"An unpleasant sensory and emotional experience associated with actual and potential tissue damage or described in terms of such damage"
Merskey et al (5)

Perhaps a more suitable interpretation may be:

"What the patient says hurts"
Oden (6)

Acute Pain

In normal development, acute pain protects us from damage as we learn what is hazardous to us. It will also limit accidental damage by causing us to withdraw from the painful stimulus and avoid it in the future. Acute pain will also prevent us from further damaging that segment by encouraging us to limit movement until it has healed. In most cases, as the injured tissue repairs itself, the pain will gradually diminish until we can again function normally.

Chronic Pain

There are occasions when the pain does not resolve on healing. Pain then is no longer a symptom of injury, but becomes a problem in its own right. This type of pain is described as chronic pain.

Injury Without Pain

Pain has a survival value, for we know that people who do not 'feel' pain may endure repeated injury that may even lead to an early death. Deficiency of the small diameter myelinated and unmyelinated C Fibres - as seen in congenital insensitivity to pain with anhidrosis - may lead to an injury such as that described by *Tachi (7)* and *Rosemberg (8)* where one third of the tongue had being bitten away by the subject. This congenital abnormality also demonstrates the functions of the C Fibres and the smaller diameter myelinated afferents, i.e. Nociception.

Hirsch (9) reported that in congenital indifference to pain, there is no abnormality in the peripheral nerves; the subject has adequate perception to painful stimuli but is indifferent to the pain. Repeated trauma may also be seen in these subjects. This further underlines how essential pain perception and normal reactions are to survival.

Pain Without Injury

Many of the patients who attend pain clinics have no history of trauma. They often attribute their problem to an incident as far back as childhood but the investigations carried out may only reveal 'degenerative changes'. These changes are often seen in asymptomatic people and may therefore be an artefact and not the root of the problem. Pain to these patients is as real as that experienced by one who has undergone surgery. The essential difference is that those who have undergone surgery will anticipate and understand their pain and will therefore expect to get better. Those without diagnosis will fear their pain, limit their mobility and continue their fruitless search for cause and cure. This group deserves the same help as those with diagnosed problems. We should not be too hasty to give these unfortunate people 'functional' or 'psychological overlay' labels.

Acute/Chronic Pain

In some diseases such as rheumatoid arthritis and osteo-arthritis, the pain may be described as chronic. In reality, the inflammation may be on going and therefore not the same as chronic pain or pain without injury.

Pain Pathways

Before discussing the ways in which TENS may effect the neuromodulation of pain, we should revise the basics of the pain pathways. Pain - known as '**nociception**' - is the neural response to painful stimuli; hence nociceptors are the peripheral receptors and peripheral primary afferents which respond to pain. It is now known that these pathways are not direct routes to the sensory cortex. Each pathway involves a framework of three ascending neurones which branch and may communicate with other neurological structures at each level.

The Nerves

Nerves are one of the means by which messages are carried around the body. When stimulated to threshold, the nerve will depolarise and an action potential will result. This wave of depolarisation or action potential sweeps along the nerve fibre at velocities in the range of 1 to 120 metres per second (m/sec) depending upon fibre type. There is not continuous flow of action potential, for when a nerve fibre has depolarised, it must re-polarise before it can be stimulated again. The time taken for re-polarisation is described as the **refractory period** during which further stimulation will not facilitate depolarisation.

The nerves carry messages about the environment e.g. temperature or our body position. This may relate to mechanical pressure such as one may feel on the soles of the feet or joint position sense. This information is carried to the Central Nervous System (CNS) where it is processed. Decisions may then be made and demands made upon muscles and viscera which are carried via efferent nerves to effect desired, or necessary changes in response to the original stimulus.

It is mainly the afferent nerves - those which carry information from the periphery to the spinal cord - which are of particular interest. Within this group, which do not only carry information relating to pain, there are three fibre types which will produce pain management when stimulated by TENS. These are the **A-beta (Aβ), A-delta (Aδ) and C fibres**.

Overview of Afferent Pathways

There are three main neurones in each chain, which form pathways for information to be carried from the periphery, via the spinal cord, to the brain, itself. There may also be small interneurones present. *Barr and Kiernan (10). See also fig' 1 on Page 16.*

For clarity, we will start at the periphery where many of the nerve endings of the afferent nerves are found, not only in the skin, but serving joint capsules, muscles, and specialist nerve endings such as Pacinian or Meissner's corpuscles.

The first neurone in the chain may be one of three types of nerve and they are described under the collective term of **first order neurones**. These nerves have their cell body within the dorsal root ganglia from which one process extends to the periphery and the second to the dorsal horn of the spinal cord. Information in the form of action potentials are carried from the periphery to the dorsal horn where the first order neurone communicates with the second order neurone via a synapse. It is this group of first order neurones which are **directly** excited by TENS. The first order neurones involved are A-beta, A-delta and C Fibres.

Second order neurones have their cell bodies in the dorsal horn of the spinal cord. These cells or neurones are excited by activity from the first order neurones and can therefore be excited indirectly by TENS. The axons of this group terminate in the thalamus where they synapse upon the cell bodies of the third order neurones. This group of neurones terminates in the sensory cortex of the brain.

Each of the three neurones in the pathway may have branches or collaterals which may synapse on the interneurones of other pathways.

Consider now that the chains of three ascending neurones, which form the pathways from the periphery of the body to the central nervous system, can be stimulated from the periphery by TENS. Also, that at each of those points where a synapse occurs in the main course of the nerves, or at one of the collaterals, neurological change may be mediated by stimulating the peripheral or first order neurones.

The peripheral nerves or first order neurones therefore provide us with a door to the CNS through which the neuromodulation of pain can be mediated. This is important, for we know that pain does not always arise from peripheral problems alone. Thalamic pain following CVA is of central origin but may still be treated from the periphery with TENS.

It is postulated that stimulating a peripheral nerve with TENS may cause changes in;
  a) the peripheral nerve itself as described by *Campbell and Taub (11)*
  b) the spinal cord as described by *Garison and Foreman (12) and Wang et al (13)*
  c) in higher centres which is evidenced by the production of endogenous opioids. *Salar et al (14), Sjölund and Eriksson (15).*

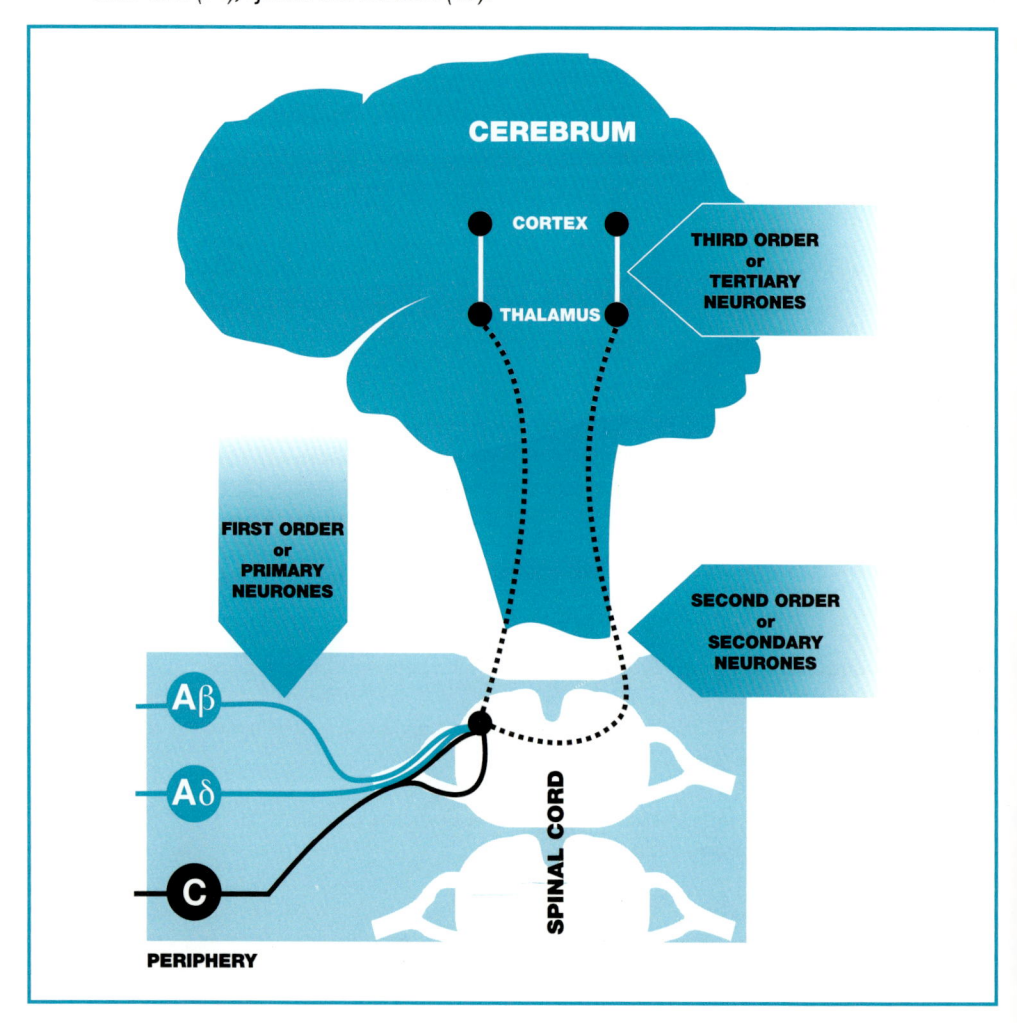

Fig 1. Ascending pathway of primary, secondary, and tertiary neurones.

Peripheral Nerves
or First Order Neurones in more detail

Remember that there are three types of first order or peripheral neurones, which are of relevance in pain management employing TENS and that each of the first order neurones will communicate with a second order neurone in the spinal cord. It is the peripheral or first order neurone where the pulsed signal produced by TENS initiates physiological changes which have analgesic implications.

The nerves involved - A-beta, A-delta and C fibres - differ in diameter, the speed or velocity at which they conduct action potentials, and the presence, or not, of an electrically insulating myelin sheath surrounding the fibres. Each carries information relating to different events in the periphery. The three types, their functions, basic physiology, and anatomy are set out below. In broad terms, the large diameter nerves have a lower threshold at which electrical stimulation will result in an action potential. The large diameter nerves also have a lower longitudinal electrical resistance and, as a result of this, conduct at a greater velocity than those nerves of a smaller diameter. The presence of a myelin sheath will further enhance conduction velocities.

Green, (16), suggests that "*The velocity of conduction in myelinated fibres is proportional to the fibre diameter; the conduction rate in metres per second (m/sec) is approximately six times the fibre diameter in microns in fibres larger than three microns*". Finally, the larger the diameter of the fibre stimulated, the more rapidly it will recover to a point where it can be further stimulated. This relates to the refractory periods.
For a more comprehensive understanding of nerve physiology the reader is directed to *Green (16) and Guyton (17)*.

1. A-Beta Nerves

A-beta nerves, the largest diameter nerves in the group under consideration are myelinated. They carry information related to proprioception (joint position sense), vibration, pressure, and touch. Due to their relatively large diameter, (up to 20 microns) and the presence of a myelin sheath, they are the fastest conducting nerves in this group at up to 120 m/sec. Williams and Warwick (18).

A-beta nerves will also respond to higher frequencies and lower intensities of stimulation. When the process of this nerve enters the spinal cord, it branches to form a collateral which is postulated to form part of the pain gate where the activity in this collateral is said to modulate 'painful traffic'. See Fig 2 on page 19. The information carried by the main trunk of the nerve is carried up to higher centres via the dorsal columns of the spinal cord. *Wells et al. (19)*.
Specific high frequency pulsed electrical stimulation of this group is suggested to produce analgesia via pain gating which is pre-synaptic inhibition of the C fibres where they synapse with the transmission cell.

2. A-Delta Nerves

This nerve type is also myelinated. The fibre diameter is less than that of the A-beta nerves and is documented as up to 5 microns. Due to the physical characteristics of this group, the conduction velocities are around 30 m/sec and the magnitude of stimulation necessary to cause an action potential is greater in this group than A-beta nerves. As this group of fibres has longer refractory periods, they will only respond to lower frequencies of stimulation. The group carries information on temperature and sharp, well-defined pain. It is the A-delta nerve which is responsible for the first or fast pain felt on injury. *Charman (20)*. It is known as a **'Nociceptor'**.

The A-delta nerves also give off collaterals within the spinal cord. The collaterals synapse with inhibitory interneurones which in turn have effects within the substantia gelatinosa. The main portion of the fibre synapses with the second order neurones which then relay the information from the A-delta fibres to higher centres where pain may be further modulated by the production of endogenous opioids. Specific low frequency or low frequency bursts of pulsed electrical stimulation of this group is suggested to produce analgesia. *See Fig.2 on page 19.*

3. C Fibres

This fibre type is unmyelinated and at 0.5 to 1.5 microns, is the smallest in diameter of the group under discussion. Conduction velocities are only 0.5 to 4 m/sec. This figure varies slightly in the different texts reviewed, however it can clearly be seen that this is the slowest conducting nerve in the group of first order neurones.

The level of stimulus required to cause an action potential in this nerve is greater than that required to stimulate the other fibre types in the group of first order neurones.

C Fibres are responsible for the slower diffuse pain which is felt up to half of one second later than that carried in A-delta fibres, (the slower or later pain is due to the slow conduction velocity). This nerve is also designated as a nociceptor. In addition to carrying information on pain the C Fibres also carry information relating to temperature and touch.

The proximal process of this nerve enters the spinal cord and synapses with a second order neurone in the posterior horn of the spinal cord. The C fibre may branch and ascend or descend up to three levels of vertebrae before synapsing. (This anatomy may be responsible for the diffuse component of later pain).

It is within the posterior horn of the spinal cord where pain gating is thought to occur. It is thought that activity in the A-beta fibres may pre-synaptically inhibit the passage of information from the C fibre to the second order neurone *(see Fig. 2 on page 19)*. If the C fibre activity is not inhibited, the information carried in C Fibres then ascends to the higher centres via the second order neurone.

In summary the peripheral or first order neurones are:

A-Beta Nerves which are large diameter, low threshold, fast conducting fibres with a low longitudinal electrical resistance to ionic current and rapid recovery times. The level of electrical stimulus that will selectively cause action potentials in these nerves is in relative terms, a **high frequency** of pulses with a **low intensity** or amplitude.

A-Delta Nerves which are approximately 25% of the diameter of A-beta nerves with a correspondingly slower conduction rate, but a higher threshold to firing, higher longitudinal electrical resistance, and a greater time for recovery. The level of electrical stimulus required to excite the A-delta fibres is of a **much lower frequency** but **higher intensity** than that required to excite the A-beta nerves.

C Fibres which are 5% or less than the diameter seen in A-beta fibres also demonstrating an **even slower** rate of conduction velocity, **higher threshold** to firing and **higher longitudinal electrical resistance** than that seen in A-delta nerves.

It follows that a lower level of stimulus is required to cause action potentials in A-beta nerves than A-delta nerves. Also that A-delta nerves will be stimulated before C Fibres. This, and the frequency dependency of response, will guide us to 'set' the TENS machine to achieve specific physiological responses in selected nerve types.

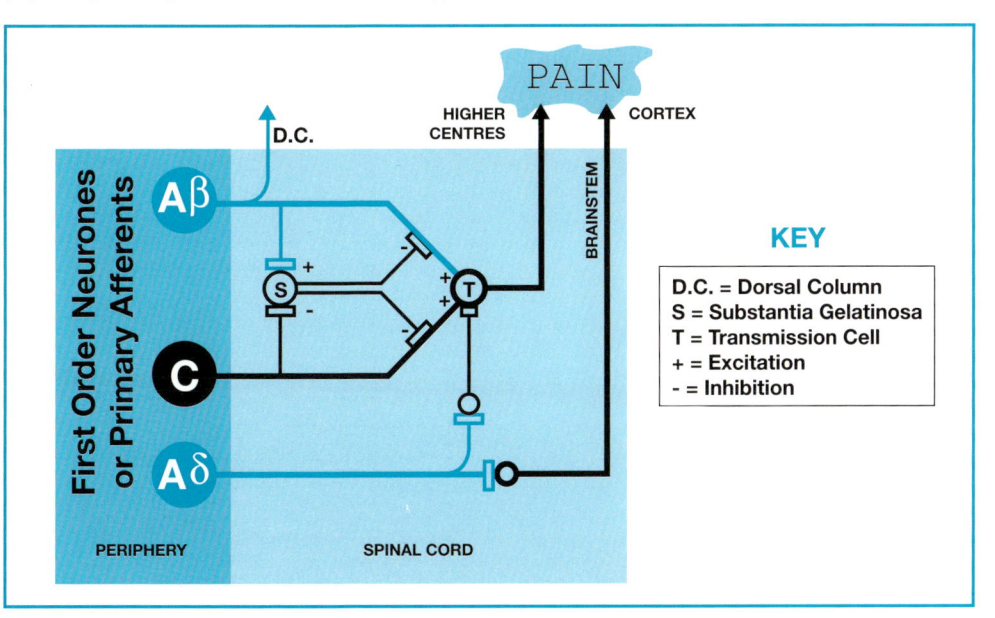

Fig 2. The Pain Gate (including A-Delta afferents)

The Nerves of the Central Nervous System

Second Order Neurones

These are the neurones on which the first order neurones synapse within the spinal cord. The second order neurones convey action potentials up to higher centres where they influence areas e.g. the thalamus and the periaqueductal grey matter. This ascending influence is thought to stimulate the production of opioids within the CNS. The opioids exhibit descending control to moderate pain.

Third Order Neurones

The final stage in the chain of neurones between the periphery of the body and the sensory cortex. It is at this level where pain comes into the conscious mind.

It may be reasonable to assume that a reduction in traffic within the pain pathways may also result in the modulation of pain.

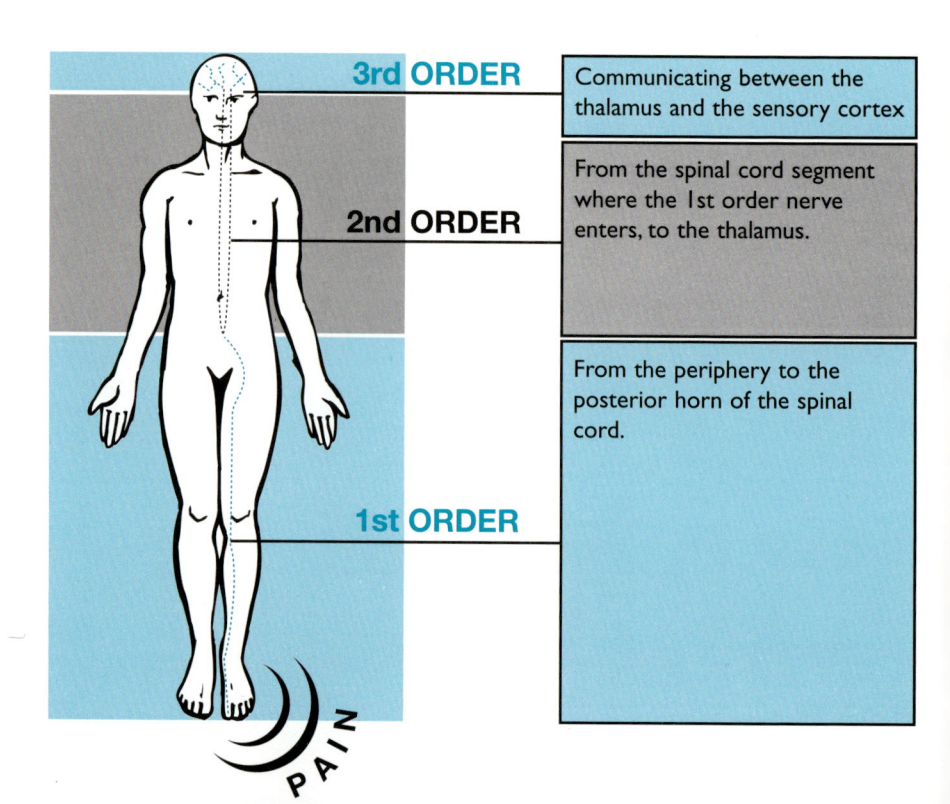

3rd ORDER — Communicating between the thalamus and the sensory cortex

2nd ORDER — From the spinal cord segment where the 1st order nerve enters, to the thalamus.

1st ORDER — From the periphery to the posterior horn of the spinal cord.

PAIN

TENS
and the Neuromodulation of Pain

It is suggested in the literature reviewed that TENS may have three modes of action upon the nervous system that may modulate pain.

1) The slowing of action potentials within the peripheral nerves thus reducing the volume of nociceptive information arriving at the spinal cord. This has been supported with experimental evidence produced by *Campbell and Taub (11)*, *Igneizi & Nyquist (21) and (22)*.

2) Activation of the Pain Gate as proposed by *Melzack and Wall (1)*. This suggests that peripheral stimulation of the large diameter afferents i.e. A-beta fibres, will cause presynaptic inhibition of the C fibres within the dorsal horn. Some investigators have questioned the presence of the pain gate, (see *reference 22 above*), however the hypothesis of pain gating does explain cause and effect in a manner which guides the successful clinical application of TENS.

3) The production of opioids has been described in many papers, e.g. *Sjölund and Eriksson (23)*, *Salar et al (14)*, and more recently by *Han and Wang (4)* who suggested that both high and low frequencies of stimulation will produce endogenous opioids. In this group of papers, it is suggested - and supported by research - that peripheral electrical stimulation of a specific type will excite higher centres (The periaqueductal grey matter is frequently mentioned as part of this system). It is in these areas that endogenous opioids are released when stimulated. It is further postulated that these neurotransmitters are responsible for the descending inhibition of nociception that occurs at segmental level.

This theory of opioid mediated analgesia is supported by experiments in which Naloxone, (a morphine antagonist), reversed analgesia produced by certain types of peripheral stimulation.

The TENS stimulation parameters which will cause the effects described above are detailed in the sections describing the TENS machine and application of TENS.

In the next section the TENS machine, its controls, and output are discussed.

The TENS Machine
It's Controls and Output

It is suggested that the reader has a TENS unit to examine when reading this next section and later to use when reading the section on 'Setting Stimulation Parameters'. The electrodes may be placed on the dorsum of the fore-arm with a minimum distance of 10cm between. Polarity will be discussed later.

As we saw earlier, the A-beta and A-delta nerves will respond to different frequencies due to different refractory (recovery) periods. The necessary magnitude of stimulation is related to the threshold at which they will depolarise and produce an action potential. It follows that we may selectively stimulate the different peripheral nerve types if we have control over these parameters.

Most, but not all of the machines that are now available, have controls which will allow (within certain ranges) adjustment of;

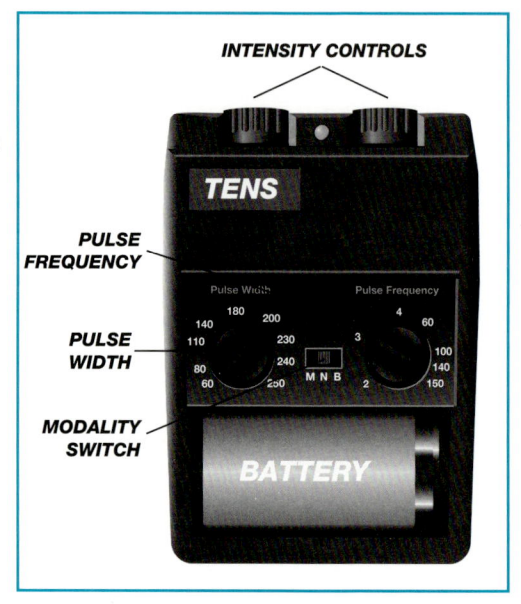

Fig 3. A Typical TENS Unit

1) **Intensity** or amplitude of each pulse which is measured in milliamps (mA) (see *Fig. 4*)
2) **Pulse Width** or duration of each pulse measured in microseconds (μ sec's)(see *Fig.4*)
3) **Frequency**, rate or number of pulses delivered per second described in Hertz (Hz)
4) **Modality** which is switchable between;
   a) **Constant** or **Normal**. Selection of this will produce a stream of pulses at a rate per second determined by the frequency selected. See *Fig 5*.
   b) **Burst** mode. Selection of this produces a group or burst of 7 to 9 pulses. This burst of pulses is repeated twice per second. See *Fig 6*.
   c) **Modulation**. In this mode the machine may automatically vary the amplitude of pulse, the frequency of pulses, or a combination of both. The manufacturers of the machines suggest that this will prevent accommodation.

A typical TENS machine and the controls of the machine are shown in Fig. 3 (above)

The parameters described on Page 22 can be combined in different ways to produce variations in signals. The combinations and their associated physiological effects will be discussed in this section.

A pulse train of the appropriate amplitude, duration and of a suitable frequency will stimulate action potentials in targeted nerves.

Melzack and Wall (24) suggest that *"nerves within about four centimetres of the skin may be stimulated by surface electrodes".*

TENS Output

Our understanding of TENS output might be helped if we first examine a single pulse (see Fig 4 below)

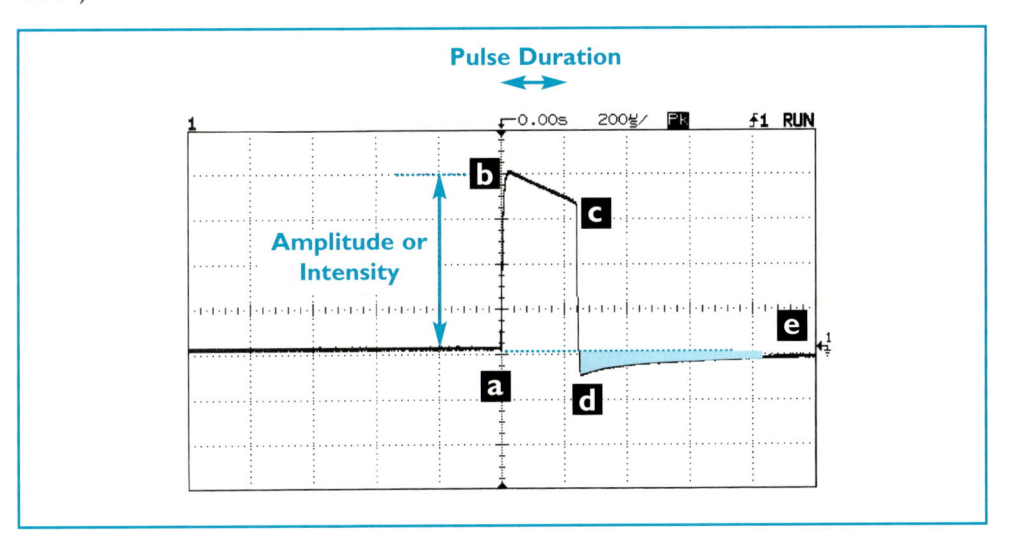

Fig 4. A Single Biphasic Pulse

The shape of the pulse is fixed and described as **biphasic**. The description 'biphasic' is applied because there are positive and negative components to the pulse. On examination of a single biphasic pulse, it can be seen that it is made up of a series of time related events.
The first component, a-b, starts at 0mA and rapidly ascends to an adjustable level of amplitude.
The second component, b-c, is the time period where the intensity level is more or less maintained. This is often described as the pulse width or pulse duration.
In the third component, c-d, the intensity falls, through zero, into a negative value.
The fourth part of the pulse, d-e, sees the negative value slowly decreasing back to zero when, in use, a further series of pulses will follow.
The area of negative current (shown hatched) helps to negate those undesirable effects of the positive current which can cause skin irritation. This biphasic pulse produces a zero net D.C. effect.

If a monophasic waveform is employed, there is a danger of a build up of chemicals between the electrode and the skin as the single pulse will result in a net positive D.C. effect. The chemicals produced may act as skin irritants.

There are two parts of each pulse, which are variable. These are:

> **Amplitude or Intensity** i.e. the amplitude of the current may be adjustable between 0 – 80 milliamps (mA) into a 500 ohm load.
>
> **Pulse Width**; the duration of each pulse is also adjustable, usually between 60 and 240 μ sec's.

Each pulse is intended to evoke an action potential in the targeted nerve. The selection of magnitude of the pulse will form one of the parameters necessary to selectively stimulate different fibre types and thus whether pain is moderated by pain gating or opioid production.

The magnitude of the stimulation could be described as a combination of amplitude and pulse width. *Walsh (3)* demonstrates graphically a strength duration curve of sensory, motor and nociceptive nerves. The strength duration curve illustrates that at low pulse duration, (10 microseconds), the amplitude of stimulation required to elicit an action potential is relatively high (> 200 mA). As the pulse duration increases, the amplitude required to produce action potentials decreases. e.g. at 200 microseconds pulse duration, most nerves will depolarise at an intensity of 80 mA.

The order in which the peripheral nerves will fire with an increasing magnitude of stimulation is also illustrated. The first to respond to an increasing stimulation are the sensory nerves of the A-beta group. These are followed by the motor nerves of A-alpha category, and finally, at higher levels of stimulation, the nociceptors of A-delta will depolarise followed, at an even higher amplitude, by the C Fibres.

Clinically, the TENS machine is not used to produce a pulse in isolation but can be adjusted via the modality switch to produce constant or normal stimulation, burst and modulation outputs.

Constant or Normal Stimulation

This is stimulation from which there is a constant stream of pulses delivered at a rate determined by the frequency or pulse rate selected before the machine is switched on (usually between 2 and 150 pulses per second). The train of pulses is delivered to the intensity selected as the machine is switched on. The amplitude is then increased to the desired level. The train of pulses will continue until the machine is switched off unless a timer is fitted to the machine. (*See Fig. 5 on page 25*)

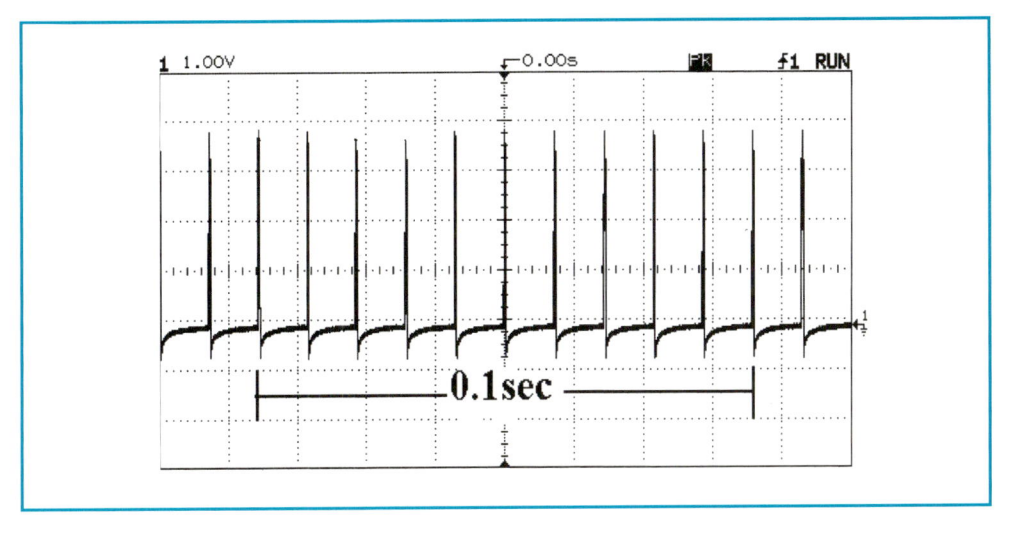

Fig 5. Constant Stimulation at 80 Hz

Burst Stimulation

Burst or 'Acupuncture Like' stimulation describes groups of 7 to 9 pulses which are produced at a rate of 2 bursts or groups per second. Again, the pulse duration and amplitude are variable but the pulse frequencies of the group and their recurrence are usually pre-set by the manufacturer. (*See Fig. 6 below*)

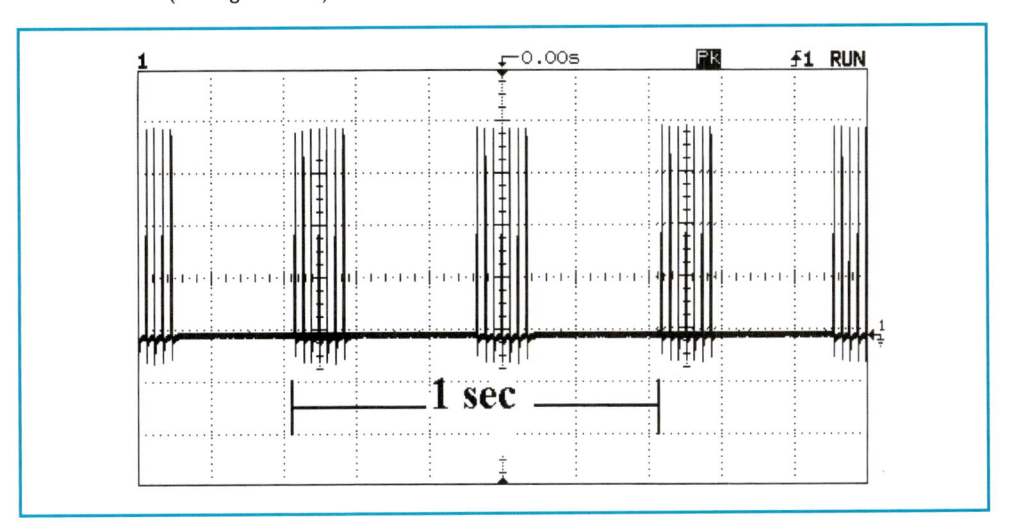

Fig 6. External Frequency of 2 Hz in Burst Stimulation.
Within each 'burst', the frequency is ± 100 Hz.

Each of the two modalities described on Page 25 are those which are most commonly used to produce pain management with TENS. A third option of **modulation** is often available on TENS units. This modality provides an automatic variation, within a range of frequency, intensity, or a combination of both. It is suggested by the manufacturers that this modality will prevent the nervous systems accommodating to TENS. Accommodation may result in a reduced reaction to stimulation and therefore negate the advantage of TENS in pain management. The writer has not reviewed any papers that support this proposition. This text will therefore concentrate only on the modalities of Constant and Burst.

Setting the TENS Machine
For Pain-Gating or Endorphin Production

To employ TENS effectively, we must first examine how the controls on the machine itself can be adjusted to facilitate one of the two methods by which the nervous system may moderate pain. In a review on endorphins and analgesia, *Sjölund and Eriksson (23)* concluded:
"There are two systems by which the CNS may be influenced by peripheral stimulation. Only one of these seems to utilise endorphins."
Later we will examine the other variables in TENS use which are part of effective pain management.

The system which appears to be independent of endorphins is suggested to be that involved in pain gating. This will be described first.

a) TENS settings necessary to facilitate pain gating

We saw earlier that closure of the pain gate is thought to be mediated by stimulation of the A-beta fibres which can be excited to threshold by a high frequency of pulses. This may be due to their relatively short refractory (recovery) period during which time they re-polarise and are susceptible to further stimulation.

The intensities at which A-beta nerves reach threshold is again relatively lower than that required to stimulate A-delta and C fibres and A-beta fibres will respond to a low level of stimulus at a high frequency of pulse delivery. The suggested parameters at which the TENS machine should be set to mediate pain management via the pain gate are detailed below.

Pulse Width or Pulse Duration.
Should be set between 100 and 200 microseconds (μ secs)

In experimental work, a pulse duration of between 100 and 900 microseconds has successfully mediated changes in dorsal horn cells, *Garison and Foreman (12)*, and peripheral nerve activity *Igneizi and Nyquist (21)*.

Sjölund and Eriksson (25) suggested that a pulse duration of 75-200 microseconds should be available for selection on all TENS machines.

As the A-beta fibres have the lowest threshold to peripheral stimulation, it is reasonable to assume that it's this group which is firing at lower pulse duration. Therefore a minimum pulse duration of 100 microseconds is suggested where the aim is to mediate pain management via the pain gate.

In a study on cold-induced pain, Johnson et al (26) employed 200 microseconds pulse duration for all modes of stimulation. The reader may consider that standardising pulse duration at 200 microseconds with all TENS treatments may be an option. This option was adopted in the pain clinic in which the author practised and has remained in place for eight years.

Frequency or Pulse Rate
Select between 80-100 Hz.

As the targeted nerves in pain gating are the large diameter A-beta afferents, we know that, due to their relatively short refractory period, only they will respond to high frequency stimulation. Sjölund and Eriksson (25) suggested 80 Hz for what they describe as conventional TENS. *Garison and Foreman (12) and Johnson (26)* further support this.

Modality
Switch to Constant

A continuous or constant stream of pulses is required to provide the 80-100 Hz stimulation necessary to selectively stimulate the A beta afferents. (See previous paragraph).

Amplitude or Intensity.

It follows that, if the aim is to stimulate the A-beta sensory nerves and stimulation from the TENS is perceived, the aim has been achieved. *Sjölund (25)* advocates that thresholds of perception of stimulation are noted and stimulation levels are then adjusted to 2-3 times that level. In clinical practice, unless calibration graphs of each machine are available, the intensity may be adjusted to a 'strong but comfortable' level of stimulation. On these settings it is not necessary to achieve visible muscle contractions. If the reader has set up the TENS as detailed, as the amplitude is increased, they will feel a buzzing or tingling sensation.

In Summary, pain gating may be mediated by;

a) Pulse Width/duration of between 100 and 200 microseconds.
b) Frequency of between 80 and 100 Hz.
c) Modality switched to Constant or Normal.
d) Amplitude or Intensity at 2-3 x threshold or a strong comfortable level of stimulation.

This type of stimulation may be perceived as a tingle or buzzing sensation

b) TENS settings necessary to facilitate the production of opioids

Early work with TENS revealed that low frequency stimulation (2-5 Hz) produced analgesia which was reversed by the introduction of Naloxone (a morphine antagonist). It was concluded from this that the induced analgesia was mediated by endogenous opioids. Later work conducted by *Sjölund and Eriksson (27) and (28)* supported that analgesia induced by low frequency stimulation was mediated by endogenous opioids.

This work also led them to develop what they described as Acupuncture-Like TENS (Burst). In a study, conventional TENS (i.e. 100 Hz with modality set at constant), was followed with acupuncture-like stimulation where useful analgesia was not achieved with the former stimulation type. *Eriksson et al (2)* found that approximately 30% of their patients had to use Burst stimulation before achieving useful analgesia.

From earlier sections the reader may recall that endogenous opioid production is the result of specific stimulation of the A-delta nerve fibres. Also, that the A-delta nerve fibre is selectively stimulated by a low frequency and high intensity pulsed current. The intensities necessary to stimulate action potentials which resulted in visible muscle contractions using low frequency continuous pulse trains were found to be uncomfortable. This led Sjölund and Eriksson to develop Burst stimulation where action potentials could be elicited at lower amplitudes or intensities of current.

The TENS settings to facilitate endogenous opioid production are set out below:

Pulse Width or Pulse Duration
Should be adjusted to a minimum of 200 microseconds (μ secs)

The production of opioids is mediated from the periphery via stimulation of the A-delta afferents. In terms of threshold, the A-delta fibres require a stimulus of greater magnitude than that employed to excite A-beta fibres. The pulse width or pulse duration is required to be at least 200 microseconds. If shorter pulse widths are employed, the amplitude needed to reach threshold will be above the range available on many TENS units.

Frequency or Pulse Rate

Most of the TENS machines that are now produced automatically set the internal and external frequencies when switched to burst mode. There are, however, some machines on which the internal frequency (see Modality on following page) can be adjusted. It is prudent therefore to adjust the frequency control to 100 Hz.

Modality
Switch to Burst

In this modality the TENS machine delivers a burst of 7-9 pulses every 0.5 sec. Each 'burst' of pulses mimics the action of a single pulse and the rate of repetition of the bursts equates to a frequency of 2 Hz. The burst signal (*see Fig 6. on page 25*) has two frequencies, an internal frequency (i.e. the burst of pulses at approximately 100 Hz), and an external frequency, at which rate each burst of pulses is repeated. As there are two bursts per second, the external frequency is at 2 Hz.

The burst of pulses avoids the necessity of the high intensities of current which are required to induce action potentials from repetitions of a single pulse at 2 Hz. It is therefore, more comfortable for the patient.

Again, the internal and external frequencies are usually pre-set during the manufacture of TENS machines.

Amplitude or Intensity.

Higher intensity levels are necessary to excite 'A' delta fibres than those used to evoke action potentials in A-beta fibres. *Eriksson and Sjölund (29)* suggest 3-5 times perception threshold or at an intensity that will evoke visible muscle contractions. However, *Librach (30)* suggests that from their observations of 4 Hz stimulation frequencies used on acupuncture points, intensity levels where the recipient feels a distinct pulsation is usually effective. This suggests that a level of stimulation where muscle contractions are not visible should be tried first. The suggestion that stimulation levels where visible muscle contractions are not necessary to produce analgesia are supported by *Johnson et al (26)*. If significant pain reduction is not achieved, higher intensities where there are visible muscle contractions may then be employed. If the reader has set up the TENS as detailed, as the amplitude is increased, they will feel a pulsating sensation.

In Summary, the production of endogenous opioids may be mediated by:

a) Pulse Width/Duration of 200 microseconds
b) Frequency; The internal and external Frequencies of burst are normally pre-set during manufacture of the machine. If you are unsure adjust to 100 Hz.
c) Modality switched to Burst
d) Initially an amplitude or intensity which is perceived as 'strong but comfortable'. If a reduction in pain is not achieved at this level of stimulation increase the intensity of stimulation until there are visible muscle contractions.

This type of stimulation may be perceived as a Pulsing or Throbbing sensation.

The selection of Conventional (Standard TENS) or Burst is discussed later in this text where it relates to specific problems. However, as a broad guide:

In practice it has been found that the majority of patients in chronic pain who respond to TENS do so with stimulation from that which mediates pain gating i.e. 80-100Hz and a Modality of Constant. If significant pain management is not achieved, the clinician may then try Burst or acupuncture-like stimulation i.e. a Modality of Burst.

Other Variables

Set Out below is a series of other variables which are external to the TENS machine but must also be considered if effective pain management is to be achieved. These are;

> 1) **Polarity of the electrodes.**
> 2) **Selecting the position of the electrodes.**
> 3) **Treatment** – How long and how often. i.e. the duration and frequency of treatments.

1) Polarity of electrodes

There are two electrodes associated with each TENS channel. These are designated;
> a) The Negative electrode or cathode whose lead connector is usually coloured black.
> b) The Positive electrode or anode. The connector is coloured red.

a) The Negative Electrode

The negative electrode is also known as the cathode and is usually coloured black. It is considered the 'active electrode', *Sjölund et al (31)*, as depolarisation of the nerve occurs beneath this electrode. It can be readily seen that the negative charge beneath the negative electrode will attract positively charged ions. This will cause changes in the relative charge of the resting potential of the underlying nerve fibre. When threshold is reached, the nerve fibre will depolarise and an action potential will result.

From what we have discussed earlier, it should be seen that the negative electrode should be placed over a nerve bundle that serves the painful area, e.g. dermatome, myotome, nerve trunk or acupuncture points.

b) The Positive Electrode

Some discussion has taken place as to whether the positive electrode should be sited proximally or distally to the negative electrode. *Mannheimer (32)* suggests that "Research should be undertaken to determine the influence of polarity as a few manufacturers suggest placing the positive electrode proximally".

The situation of polarity is further clouded if one reads the chapter by *Sjölund et al (31)* in which the reader is advised to place the negative electrode proximally when using conventional TENS (80-100 Hz with a modality of constant). However, if stimulating with acupuncture like TENS is employed (Burst), Sjölund then suggests that the negative electrode should be placed distally to stimulate motor neurones which will activate muscle contractions and powerful indirect deep afferent flow.

Walsh (3) describes the anodal effects (that of the positive electrode) as hyperpolarisation which may change the membrane potential towards a more negative value. It is suggested later in the same text that hyperpolarisation may impede the conduction of action potentials, therefore the cathode should be placed proximally and the anode distally.

The implications from the papers reviewed are that:

> Hyperpolarisation may create a block to the conduction of an action potential…

> …or nerve fibres may require a greater magnitude of stimulation to continue to affect depolarisation to threshold and therefore the production of action potentials.

The pain clinic in which the author practised evolved what was called **dermatomal stimulation**. This was an attempt to achieve accurate stimulation of the affected segment or painful areas (see the later section on electrode position). In this arrangement the active or negative electrode (black) was placed distally, usually over the dermatome associated with the pain or just proximal to the pain. The positive (red) electrode was placed paravertebrally over the nerve root which served that dermatome.

Initially polarity reversals were tried with the individuals who were not responding to TENS. The changes in polarity did not reveal any significant changes in the pain management of these individuals. Following this period, the orientation of polarity followed by the clinic was maintained as;

> **Negative** electrode (cathode) distally
> **Positive** electrode (anode) proximally

Annual audit of patient notes was commenced in 1992. This demonstrated a significant improvement in linear pain scales of between 60% in 1992 and 80% in 1997/98 of those patients referred for TENS trials.

In 1992, the writer carried out a small scale study (unpublished) to determine if anodal block was evident in TENS use. In this study, the intensities necessary to evoke both paraesthesia and visible muscle contractions were established for each polarity. The study failed to demonstrate a significant difference between the intensities recorded for each polarity which were necessary to produce paraesthesia from TENS stimulation or that required to evoke visible muscle contractions. The levels of intensity were recorded from the amplitude control of the TENS machine. Although the same machine and channel were used throughout the trial, this is a crude method of measurement. It would be necessary to repeat the trial using methods of measurement that will stand up to scrutiny.

The studies reviewed, which describe anodal block or hyperpolarisation, involved the dissecting out of nerves which were then electrically stimulated by adjacent electrodes.
Casey and Blick (33), Mendell and Wall (34).

As the body acts as a volume conductor, the reactions recorded in the studies above may not apply in the clinical use of TENS. The targeted nerves may lie some distance from the stimulating electrodes or be surrounded by other structures which may conduct current away from the targeted nerve. It may then be difficult to predict what the actual effects of, or level of current is actually acting upon the targeted nerve.

In addition to the above, the hyperpolarisation which may occur beneath the anode will have a duration of the same time period of the cathode. In a situation where the pulse duration is set to 200 μ secs (0.2 ms) and the frequency is adjusted to 80 Hz, the time period between each pulse will be around 12 ms. The ratio of the interlude between pulses to pulse duration will be of the order of 60:1. This may be relevant when one considers that the action potential takes a relatively long time to travel from cathode to anode. The condition where anodal block may take place may require that the action potential must pass under the anode in a manner which is synchronous to cathodal polarisation. The question of polarity is still an area where further research is indicated.

In summary:

> **In the clinical application of TENS, if the TENS machine is first used with the electrodes in an 'anode proximal to cathode' orientation and significant improvement is not evident, the clinician may simply reverse the polarity and re-assess the effectiveness of TENS.**

2) Selecting the position of the electrodes

From earlier sections in this text, it may be seen that one of the areas to attempt TENS stimulation may be over the nerve trunks which supply the area in which the pain is felt. The reader may already be familiar with the necessary anatomy to achieve this. However, for those who require vision or revision of neuro-anatomy there are many books which cover this subject. e.g. *Williams and Warwick (18), Lockhart Hamilton & Fyfe (35),* and a colour atlas by *McMinn et al (36).*

A further and simpler method of selecting electrode positions relates to the dermatomes. The area of skin supplied by afferent nerve fibres from a single nerve root is described as a **dermatome**. It follows that if pain is felt in a particular dermatome, stimulation of that dermatome and its associated nerve root may stimulate the appropriate afferent nerves. (A section of dermatome maps is included on pages 34 and 35). It is suggested that the reader identifies the dermatome in which the pain or referred pain lies and places the cathode (black) just proximal to the pain. The anode (red) may then be placed paravertebrally at the level of the nerve root. (A section on locating vertebrae is included on pages 34 and 35). This method of electrode site selection may also be applied to the **myotomes**.

Mannheimer (32) suggests that electrode sites may be tried at;
    a) Acupuncture, motor or trigger points
    b) The location of greatest tenderness or pain
    c) Distant or contralateral sites
    d) Specific dermatomes or spinal segmental levels
    e) Superficial points along peripheral nerves.
    f) Linear pathways.

A method of probing for superficial points of nerves is described by *Berlant (37)* who also noted that the points producing the greatest degree of radiating paraesthesia were also major acupuncture points.

In a study of electrode placements and stimulating parameters, *Wolf et al (38)* placed electrodes initially at the site of pain, along the peripheral nerve proximally to the site of pain or paravertebrally at the related nerve root(s). If these placements failed to produce adequate pain relief, trigger or motor points were tried on contralateral homologous or remote sites. However, this study failed to find a precise correlation between stimulating procedures, electrode placements and pain relief.

Walsh (3) analysed several clinical and experimental studies and concluded that acupuncture points are apparently effective and increasingly popular electrode placement sites. Also that, "*The overwhelmingly positive results from studies using acupuncture points suggest that they should be at least considered*".

In summary:

> **Electrode sites** should relate to the nerves that serve the painful area. It is suggested by the writer that a starting point for electrode placement may be within the dermatome that pain is felt. Place the cathode within the dermatome in which the pain is described, just proximal to the pain. The anode may be placed paravertebrally over the nerve root related to that dermatome on the same side. If significant pain management is not achieved, placements over myotomes, acupuncture points or nerve bundles may be tried.
>
> There may also be occasions when placing electrodes each side of a painful joint may help. eg. the front and back of a painful shoulder. (See *Fig. 7 below*)

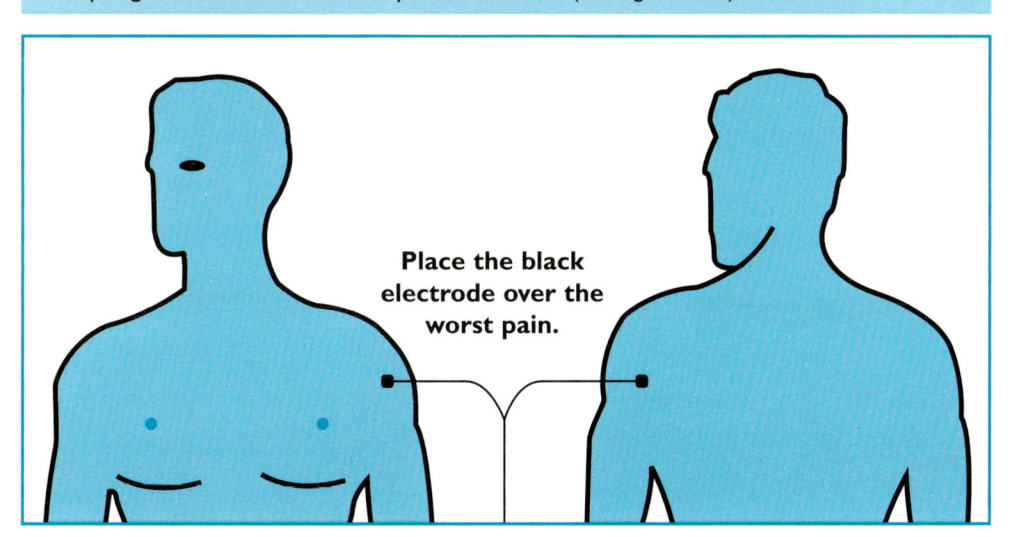

Place the black electrode over the worst pain.

Fig 7. Example of placing electrodes either side of a painful joint

Locating Vertebrae

The spinal column is divided into regions to simplify identification. Those that are of interest to us are the cervical spine (C1-7), the thoracic spine (T1-12), and the lumbar spine (Ll-5).

Cervical Spine
If you drop your chin towards your chest, a prominence will rise on the back of your neck. This is the spinous process of C7 and is usually found approximately level with the tops of the shoulders. It is the most prominent of the cervical vertebrae. Once C7 has been located it is a simple matter to palpate and count up to the desired level. It should be remembered that the nerve roots associated with numbered cervical vertebrae lie above the vertebra up to C7. The C8 nerve root lies below C7.

Thoracic Spine
The vertebra lying below C7 is T1. T7 is found by placing the arms by the sides. If the lowest points of the scapulae are palpated for, T7 will be found at the same level on the midline. The other thoracic vertebrae may be identified by counting up or down from these points. The thoracic nerve roots lie below each of the numbered vertebrae, e.g. the nerve root T2 lies between T2 and T3.

Lumbar Spine
Place your hands on your waist and palpate firmly down until you encounter the uppermost brim of the pelvis. Once identified, this lies at the same level as L4, again found on the midline. Palpate each spinous process up to identify L3-1 or palpate one spinous process down to identify L5. The lumbar nerve roots also lie below each numbered vertebrae. eg. the L3 nerve root lies between L3 and L4.

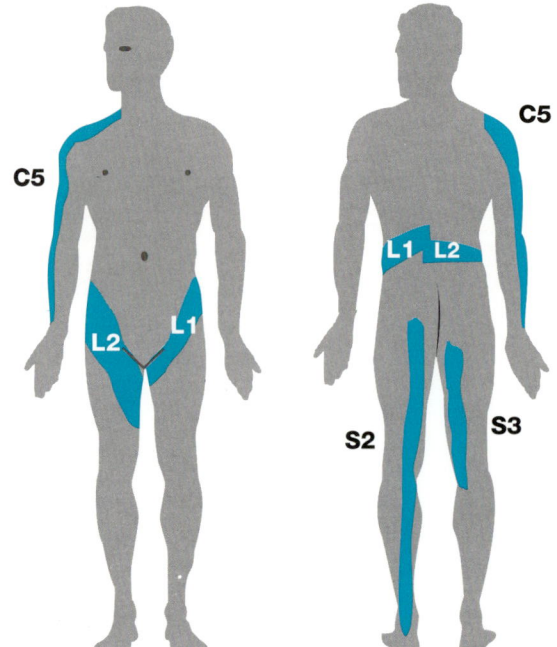

KINGS Professionals' Guide to TENS

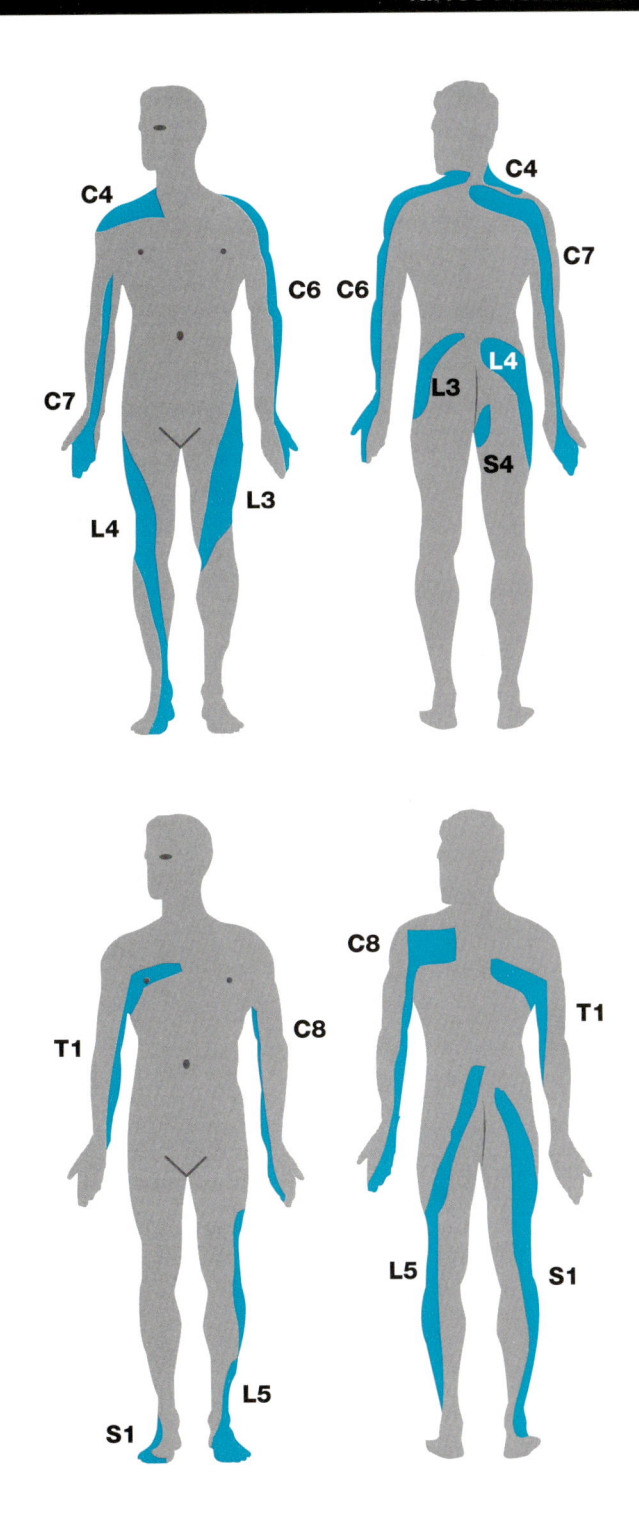

3) Treatments: How long and how often?
The duration and frequency of treatments

In 1978 *Mannheimer (32)* suggested that the most effective duration and frequency of treatment may require further research.

Duration
The necessary duration of treatment in the papers reviewed have been suggested to be 15 minutes to continuous stimulation. *Librach (30) Sjölund (31) and Szeto and Nyquist (39).*

In a study examining CSF samples post stimulation with TENS, *Han et al (40)* found significant changes in opioid levels following 30 minutes of TENS stimulation. *Eriksson (2)* found the induction time of analgesia in conventional TENS to be 2-10 minutes where in acupuncture like or burst TENS, onset was between 20 and 30 minutes. In the last two studies sighted, it may be seen that the lower point in treatment duration may be greater than 30 minutes.
In a study on electrode placements and stimulating parameters, *Wolf (38)* employed stimulation times of 30-45 minutes for 3-5 treatments. In his discussion, it was suggested that the future use of TENS should concentrate on longer duration and more frequent treatment sessions.

Frequency of Treatments
Again, there is a wide range of suggestions as to the best frequency rate for treatment; however, many suggest 3-4 treatments per day. *Librach (30)* suggests that patients should be advised to use TENS on an 'as necessary' basis with breaks between treatments determined by the level of pain control. Thus, if there is good pain relief for two hours after a treatment, the treatments should be two hours apart.

The treatment times should be of sufficient duration to stimulate analgesia of significant magnitude and duration without causing unnecessary side effects. The frequency of treatment repetition should be dictated by the results one achieves. Most workers suggest 3-4 times daily. The frequency and duration of treatment selected at the outset of treatment is just a starting point. You will be guided by the re-assessments of your patient and their reaction to TENS.

In summary:

a) Treatment duration may start at 60-90 min's and be adjusted up or down as indicated by results. (The first treatment should be of a shorter duration to observe for adverse reactions). Treatments where burst is employed at an intensity which evokes muscle contractions should be limited to 20-30 minutes.

b) Treatment frequency may commence at 4 times per day and, again, be adjusted as necessary.

The Pain Gate
Versus Endorphin Production

As pain gating is postulated to be mediated by the stimulation parameters of Constant, 80-100 Hz and endorphin production mediated by Burst, the question the reader may ask is;

Which modality do I use first?

One may consider that the stimulation parameters that yield the greatest degree of success should be tried first, not only for the patient's sake, but to reduce the time and therefore the cost involved in treating each individual.

Eriksson et al (2) suggest that 30% of the patients in their long-term study had to use burst to achieve useful analgesia. The conclusion that we may draw from this is that, of those successfully treated, 70% responded to Constant 80-100 Hz stimulation.
In a review of TENS, *Lundeberg (41)* described High TENS (Constant 80-100 Hz) as 50% successful in treating peripheral neuropathies, joint pain, skeletal, neurogenic and stump pain. He goes on to describe Low TENS as of *"special value where cutaneous sensitivity is impaired"*. Conversely, low frequency TENS of 4 Hz, (equates to Burst), is recommended over acupuncture points by *Librach and Rapson (30)* in their study into pain relief in palliative care. The opposite view is taken by *Johnson et al (26)* who achieved the greatest statistical reliability in producing significant analgesia with 80 Hz constant stimulation. This was in volunteers with cold induced pain. *Sjölund et al (31)* simplify the question for us by suggesting that Acupuncture-like TENS (Burst) should be utilised when Constant stimulation fails.

In summary:

> As a general rule, the stimulation parameters which are suggested to mediate pain gating i.e. mode of Constant, frequency of 80-100 Hz, pulse duration 100-200μ seconds should be tried first. Where the above fails to produce significant pain management, the modality of burst and a pulse duration of 200μ seconds should be tried.

Indications for Treatment

The papers reviewed describe successful treatment in conditions ranging from angina pectoris, *Marshall (42)*, to osteoarthritic knees, *Grimmer (43)*. It would perhaps be simpler to describe the pain problems that TENS is **not** indicated in attempting to treat!

Other than pain arising from deep visceral structures where it is difficult to stimulate the appropriate nerve supply and pain arising from the mass itself in cancer, the clinician may consider that an attempt to treat any of the problems presented is indicated.

The goal of treatment with those in chronic pain is to produce analgesia. When treating with TENS, the most likely outcome will be a significant reduction in pain for significant periods of time. The result therefore is not a cure but temporary analgesia. If the patient is prepared to accept this outcome as a positive result, a trial of TENS may be indicated.

Following diagnosis, (where possible), and an assessment of the patient, Sjölund suggests that the clinician should be aware of three points.

> **a) The origin of the pain**
> **b) The maintaining factors**
> **c) Observed pain behaviour**

a) The origin of the pain
This may be neuropathic or nociceptive. Neuropathic pain may involve any of the peripheral nerve injuries, insults to the spinal cord or those of higher centres such as thalamic pain, sometimes seen post CVA. Nociceptive pain includes any of the musculoskeletal, vascular or referred pains. There may be an overlap between neuropathic and neurogenic pain due to pathology or injury; however, all may respond to TENS.

b) The maintaining factors
Among maintaining factors, there is a phenomenon known as 'wind up'. This occurs when the C fibres respond in an increasing magnitude to each successive stimulus. This can cause a temporary increase in pain when first using TENS. The information given to the patient pre-TENS trial should include this fact. TENS, due to the effects of stimulation on C fibres, also reduces wind up in the longer term. (See page 11). Other maintaining factors include poor posture, the unnecessary limiting of movement and obesity.

c) Observed pain behaviour
Pain Behaviour requires modification via a Pain Management Programme and is not directly reduced by TENS treatments. *Sjölund (31)* suggests that TENS should be used as part of a multi-modal therapy.

Each of the factors described will prevent the patient from leading a 'normal life' and must all be addressed to lead the patient away from dysfunction. TENS has direct effects on the first two but should form part of a combined treatment, which may include counselling, in the third.

In summary:

> The only exclusion criteria for trying TENS **may** be one of attempting to treat patients with a positive psychiatric evaluation and possible psychogenic pain as *Eriksson (2)* found that this group, as a rule did not respond to TENS treatments. One must be wary of the term 'psychological overlay', which may be found in the notes of many patients suffering from chronic pain. This assertion is often indicative of the clinician's frustration in their failure to resolve the patients problem rather than the actual mental state of the person involved.

Notes, Assessment and Re-assessment

The keeping of notes is a legal requirement. There are other compelling reasons to keep accurate notes for, among the many people in pain, there are those whose only measure of successful treatment is complete freedom from pain. The notes then provide objective evidence to the patient of any improvement and also guide us in our adjustments of the variables in TENS.

The difficulties associated with assessing pain have led to the development of such devices as the 'McGill Pain Questionnaire' and variations of the same. *Reading (44)* described the McGill Questionnaire as a valid, reliable instrument to measure pain experience. It was produced in a shortened form but still requires a significant amount of time to complete and analyse. This has led to this valuable tool being ignored in many clinics.

In an attempt to produce a valid and easily used assessment and re-assessment tool we developed a proforma assessment and review form in the pain clinic where the writer practiced. A copy of this may be found at the end of the section. This may be photocopied and enlarged to A4 size by the reader if they wish.

The front sheet includes the usual sections to identify the patient and referring clinician, social history, previous medical history and history of presenting complaint. A diagnosis and what the patient perceived as the main problem are also recorded. There follows two columns of factors that many of the patients had felt were affected by their pain before and after a trial of TENS. These include;

a) The average total hours of sleep achieved each night
b) How many times their sleep is disturbed
c) A number between 1-10 relating to a linear pain scale reading where 0 = pain free and 10 = the worst possible pain
d) A list of the pain relieving medication and doses that they are taking
e) A description of a level of function that the patient felt is affected by their pain

The above are recorded on assessment, review and on discharge when comparisons can be made.

The first section is followed by a body plan where the patient may illustrate the areas of pain. A description and identification of the TENS machine itself follows. The settings of the TENS machine and recommended levels of use are also recorded.

Sections for reviews are also provided, each of which provides a record of;

   a) Review of the Linear Pain Scale
   b) A subjective comment
   c) Current levels of function relating to that recorded on initial assessment
   d) Current sleep pattern
   e) Analysis of any changes in symptoms

There follows a section in each review where any changes made in stimulation parameters may be recorded. Provision is made for five reviews. Additional sheets of review proforma should be made available when necessary.

It is not suggested that the assessment proforma included is a solution to pain assessment and re-assessment when using TENS. It is hoped that the reader may find it useful as a starting point in setting up their own note system tailored to the needs of the service that they provide to their patients.

TENS ISSUE

NAME

Address

Tel. No.

Social History

PMH

HPC

Diagnosis

Main Problem

DOB

1st Apt.

Discharge Date

Issue TENS

Return TENS

Consultant

Clinician

ON ASSESSMENT

Hours sleep

Broken x

LPS min

LPS max

HAD pre Rx

Function

Drug Hx

ON DISCHARGE

Hours sleep

Broken x

LPS min

LPS max

HAD post Rx

Function

Drug Hx

Total Patient Contacts

DNA

UTA

Purchase TENS

Long Term Loan

Discharged. from Service

Consultant Review

Safety Check

TENS Issued on

Serial No.

C **B** **M**

Freq **Hz** **PW** μs

Applitude **L** **R**

Use **mins** **Freq daily**

Signed:

FIRST TENS REVIEW

DATE _____   Hours slept _____   Broken x _____

LPS Min _____   LPS Max _____   Function _____

Changes in Drug x _____

TREATMENT CHANGES

[ ] B [ ] M [ ]

Frequency _____ Hz

Pulse Width _____ μs

Electrode position (as body plan) _____

LEVELS OF USE

Mins _____   Freq _____

Comments _____

Signed _____

....

SECOND TENS REVIEW

DATE _____   Hours slept _____   Broken x _____

LPS Min _____   LPS Max _____   Function _____

Changes in Drug x _____

TREATMENT CHANGES

[ ] B [ ] M [ ]

Frequency _____ Hz

Pulse Width _____ μs

Electrode position (as body plan) _____

LEVELS OF USE

Mins _____   Freq _____

Comments _____

Signed _____

THIRD TENS REVIEW

DATE _____ **Hours slept** _____ **Broken x** _____

LPS Min _____ **LPS Max** _____ **Function** _____

Changes in Drug x _____

TREATMENT CHANGES

C [ ]   B [ ]   M [ ]

Frequency _____ Hz

Pulse Width _____ μs

Electrode position (as body plan)
_____

LEVELS OF USE

Mins _____   **Freq** _____

Comments _____

Signed _____

FOURTH TENS REVIEW

DATE _____ **Hours slept** _____ **Broken x** _____

LPS Min _____ **LPS Max** _____ **Function** _____

Changes in Drug x _____

TREATMENT CHANGES

C [ ]   B [ ]   M [ ]

Frequency _____ Hz

Pulse Width _____ μs

Electrode position (as body plan)
_____

LEVELS OF USE

Mins _____   **Freq** _____

Comments _____

Signed _____

ADDITIONAL COMMENTS

Anti-Emisis

Work on peripheral stimulation with acupuncture carried out by *Dundee et al (46)*, where the P6 acupuncture point was stimulated in patients undergoing minor gynaecological operations, markedly reduced the incidence of vomiting and nausea in the first six post-operative hours.

Nausea may be post-operative, that seen in the early stages of pregnancy, or caused by chemotherapy. See *Al-Sadi et al (47) and Dundee et al (46)*.

Later work carried out by *McMillan and Dundee (48)* demonstrated that TENS stimulation over the P6 acupuncture point also had a significant effect in reducing nausea post chemotherapy treatment.

This point Circulation 6 is described below.

Circulation 6: Lies upon the anterior surface of the forearm, two-inches above the distal wrist crease between the tendons of Palmaris Longus and Flexor Carpi Radialis.

If TENS is to be used to stimulate Circulation 6, the black (active) electrode should be placed over the point. The red electrode may then be placed either over the Thenar Eminence or mid-forearm, anterior aspect.

The TENS machine may be set as follows:

 a) **Pulse Width at 200 microseconds**
 b) **Modality set to Burst**
 c) **Frequency set to 100 Hz**

Stimulate for between five minutes and one hour. Repeat two hourly. *McMillan and Dundee (48)* suggest low frequencies of 10-15 Hz for five minutes every two hours.

Side Effects

1) The main side effects seen in TENS use are related to the dermis and may involve:

   a) An electrical burn. This can be avoided by taking care that the skin sites selected possess normal sensation, the duration of treatments are not unnecessarily long and the intensities of stimulation are not excessive. Careful observation of the electrode sites in the early stages of treatment is advised.

   b) Contact allergies. These may relate to the gel used as an interface between the electrode and the skin, carbon rubber electrodes or the adhesive tape used to fix the electrodes in place. These problems can, in most cases, be resolved by changing to hypoallergenic self-adhesive electrodes. Where the allergy continues, the causative agent must be identified and an alternative found. e.g. Karaya gel may be used as the interface between electrode and skin or micropore tape used for fixing electrode to skin.

2) TENS may cause an increase in pre-existing lymphoedema.

3) Headaches may result from stimulation using certain parameters. Some patients describe the headache as 'hangover like' in nature. The stimulation responsible for this phenomenon varies between patients. This problem can usually be resolved by reducing the pulse duration (where the new level will continue to excite the targeted nerve type). Changes in the other stimulation parameters may also resolve this problem.

4) Hypotension may result from electrode placements around the cervical spine.

5) There may be a temporary increase in pain due to the 'wind up' phenomenon.

Not a side effect of TENS but one that may diminish the effectiveness of TENS may be the ingestion of caffeine. In an investigation into its effects, *Marchand et al (45)* administered volunteers orally with either 200mg of caffeine or a placebo before subjecting them to thermally induced pain. This group of workers found that the analgesic effects of TENS were abolished in those subjects who had ingested caffeine. They concluded that *"One cup of coffee contains between 60-125 mg of caffeine; thus, two or three cups of coffee could block the effect of TENS"*.

Choosing Equipment

The TENS Machine

There is a myriad of TENS machines available on today's market, some of which do not produce an output of signal that will satisfactorily stimulate both A β and A δ nerve fibres.

Pulse Duration

We have seen earlier that a pulse duration of 200 μ sec's is necessary to depolarise A δ nerve fibres where A β fibres will respond to a Pulse Duration of 100 m sec's at the levels of amplitude accessible on many of the available machines. It follows that the available range of selectable pulse duration should be at least 100-200 μ sec's. The range usually seen is around 60-250 μ sec's.

Modality

A number of the available machines only possess the modality of 'Continuous' stimulation. This is also referred to as 'Normal' or 'Constant' by some manufacturers. Although Continuous Stimulation is entirely satisfactory for exciting A β nerves at a frequency of 80-100 Hz, some patients may that find 2 Hz continuous stimulation and a pulse duration of 200 μ sec's, which are necessary to stimulate the A δ nerve fibres, uncomfortable. The modality of 'Burst', also referred to as 'acupuncture-like' stimulation, is a desirable feature as this modality will cause depolarisation at lower amplitudes than those required at 2 Hz with constant modality.

The modality of 'Modulation' may also be found on some of the available machines. The suppliers and manufacturers suggest that this feature will reduce the accommodation that may occur in TENS use. The writer has not reviewed any papers to support this proposition. The available information would indicate that the facility to switch between Continuous and Burst types of stimulation is an important feature.

Frequency

Where the aim is to stimulate pain gating via the A β nerves, a frequency of 80 to 100 Hz must be available. Even though some patients may find 2 Hz Continuous stimulation uncomfortable, there are those who prefer to employ this frequency in order to facilitate endorphin production. Those machines that have adjustable frequency usually have a range of 2-150 Hz available.

Amplitude

This is normally measured in milliamps (mA). The manufacturer will normally state the load at which the output has been measured. Many still use a 500 Ω load. *Walsh (3)* suggests a 1000 Ω load which is approximately taken to represent the average skin-electrode impedance.
The strength-duration curve of stimulation amplitude against pulse duration *Sjölund (25)* shows that all peripheral nerves will depolarise at 80 mA with a pulse duration of 200 μ sec's. The maximum available amplitude on many machines is of the order of 80 mA into a 500 Ω load.

A final point on the control of amplitude relates to the advancement of the amplitude control. This should see a gradual or linear increase in output between each of the graduations. On many of the TENS tested by the writer, the relationship between the numbers on the control knob and actual output were not linear. This reinforces the suggestion by *Walsh (3)* that calibration graphs for each machine should be recorded during the testing of TENS before clinical use. The graphs may then be at hand to record the amplitudes used by each patient.

Controllability or User-friendliness

One must bear in mind the dexterity of the patients who will use the machine away from the support of the clinic. Even though the internal controls may be set by the clinician, the patient will still be required to turn the machine on and off and to adjust the amplitude of the machine. The controls must therefore be accessible without being so prominent that they can be accidentally increased.

In summary.

> The machines purchased should have adjustments of:
> a) Pulse duration between at least 100-200 μ sec's.
> b) Selectable modalities of 'Continuous' and 'Burst'
> c) An adjustable frequency with a minimum range of 2-150 Hz.
> d) A gradually adjustable amplitude of 0-80 mA into at least a 500 Ω load

Other Equipment

Lead Wires

These are normally around one metre in length and are easily separated to allow electrodes to be placed some distance apart. The terminals to the electrodes should be colour coded so that the anode and cathode can be identified.

Electrodes.

From personal experience of pre and post lumbar micro-discectomy, accurately placing electrodes and fixing them with adhesive tape on the lumbar region without assistance is quite difficult. The highly flexible self-adhesive electrodes are easier to place and have a much longer useable life than their earlier predecessors.

There may still be a place for carbon rubber electrodes and gel to be used in trials held before the issue of TENS. However, it should be remembered that carbon rubber electrodes also have a limited life span. Even though they appear to be serviceable, after three months the electrical resistance they offer increases. The new re-usable self-adhesive electrodes may also last three months or more.

In summary:

> Even though self-adhesive re-usable electrodes may seem expensive when compared to carbon rubber, the ease of application and reduced incidence of allergic response may make them a choice of preference.

KINGS Professionals' Guide to TENS

Information for Patients

Supporting information for any course of treatment is important. It offers reassurance to the patients when problems arise and answers many of the questions that patients may forget to ask during assessment and review sessions.

There follows a sample of the leaflet provided to the patients in the pain clinic where the writer practised. This was developed from the common questions asked over a number of years. The reader may wish to use this sample as a guide and further develop it to suit the particular service that they offer.

TENS Information Booklet Sample

YOU MUST NOT USE A TENS MACHINE IF YOU ARE FITTED WITH A PACEMAKER

IF YOU ARE IN THE FIRST TWELVE WEEKS OF PREGNANCY, YOU MUST ONLY USE TENS ON THE ADVICE OF YOUR CLINICIAN.

YOU SHOULD NOT USE A TENS OVER BROKEN OR DAMAGED SKIN.

DO NOT HAVE YOUR TENS SWITCHED ON WHEN DRIVING OR OPERATING MACHINERY

This booklet is intended to give you a broad view of **TENS** and how it should be used. Spend a little time reading this, it is intended to support the verbal information given to you by your consultant and clinicians.

WILL 'TENS' CURE MY PAIN?
TENS or Transcutaneous Electrical Nerve Stimulation, is not a 'cure-all'. If you fall within the 80% or so of people who are helped by TENS, you will experience a reduction in pain rather than a cure. This reduction in pain will provide you with an opportunity to gradually increase what you can do.

HOW DO I FEEL PAIN?
The sensory part of pain involves a series of impulses being carried along the nerve fibres in the limbs and body. The nerve fibres then enter the spinal cord and communicate with a further group of nerves which carry the pain signals up to the brain where the signal is converted into the sensation of pain.

CAN THE PAIN BE REDUCED?
Yes, if in some way the pain signal can be slowed or reduced, then the pain felt would also be reduced.

HOW WILL TENS REDUCE MY PAIN?
When anyone bangs their head or elbow, they instinctively rub the sore part. This 'rubbing' causes a great deal of activity in the thickest nerve fibres. When this information reaches the spine, it is treated as 'more important' than the painful impulses which are carried in the smaller nerve fibres. The pain in turn is lessened.

TENS works in a very similar way in as much as it electrically stimulates the thicker nerves. This stimulation in turn 'blocks' some of the pain.

IS THIS 'BLOCKING' OF PAIN THE ONLY WAY THAT TENS CAN REDUCE MY PAIN?
No. The TENS unit can also be adjusted to stimulate the body to produce its own pain-killing chemicals, (endorphins or endogenous opioids). Again, this is not a cure, but pain management.

WHERE DO I PUT THE ELECTRODES?
When you are loaned a TENS unit, you will be shown where to place the sticky electrodes which carry the current from the TENS unit - via thin wires - to the skin. The current will be felt as a tingling or pulsing sensation under the electrodes.

CAN I CHANGE THE POSITION OF THE ELECTRODES?
No. The position of these electrodes is very important. Your clinician will place them over the nerves involved in transmitting your pain. When you replace the electrodes each morning, it is important that you put them back in the same place. (A body plan is included in the booklet to guide you).

DOES MY SKIN NEED ANY SPECIAL CARE WHEN I USE TENS?
You must wash the area of skin where the electrodes go at least once a day with soap and water, rinse and dry well. This is best done first thing in the morning before you position your electrodes.

CAN I USE BODY LOTIONS OR CREAMS WHERE THE ELECTRODES GO?
No. They will prevent the electrodes from sticking to your skin. They will also shorten the life of the electrode.

HOW LONG DO I LEAVE THE ELECTRODES ON?
Once positioned, leave the electrodes in place all day rather than putting them on and taking them off each time you use your TENS during the day. However, if you have any skin problems using TENS, you may need to remove the electrodes after each treatment.

DO THE ELECTRODES NEED ANY SPECIAL CARE?
Yes. When not in use overnight, stick them back onto the plastic film supplied with the electrodes. Do not stick the electrodes face to face as this will destroy them. If the electrodes lose some of their 'stickiness', try moistening the surface with a few drops of water.

HOW DO I SET THE TENS MACHINE?
The TENS machine will be set for you by your clinician. You may adjust the intensity (strength) of the machine, but the internal controls should only be adjusted by your clinician.

HOW LONG DO I USE MY TENS FOR EACH DAY?
Attach the lead wires to the machine and switch on for between one and one and a half hours. This can be repeated up to four times a day, giving a maximum total of six hours a day.

WHAT WILL I FEEL?
Gradually increase the intensity until you can feel a strong but comfortable tingling (you may only feel this through one of the pair of electrodes - this is not unusual).
After twenty minutes or so, you may not be able to feel the tingling. If this is the case, gradually increase the intensity until you can feel a comfortable tingle again.

SHOULD I STOP TAKING MY MEDICATION WHEN I'M USING TENS?
No. Continue with your medication until directed otherwise.

SHOULD I REST WHEN I'M USING MY TENS?
No. The whole idea in making the TENS portable is to allow you to move around and to help you regain 'normal activity'. The more that you move, the more that pain will be inhibited. You should aim to gradually increase your present level of activity.

WILL I GET BETTER PAIN RELIEF IF I GRIT MY TEETH AND TURN THE MACHINE UP HIGH?
No. If you turn the machine up too high, you may start to stimulate the nerves which carry the painful impulses or cause skin irritation. It is important that you only turn up your machine so that you can feel a strong, comfortable tingle unless your clinician directs you otherwise.

WHAT CAN I EXPECT?
It may be up to 20 minutes before you experience any reduction in pain. When you switch your machine off, it may be some time before your pain returns to its former intensity. This is called 'carry over'.

WHAT DO I DO IF MY SKIN BECOMES SORE WHEN USING TENS
If you have any skin problems when using TENS or any problems with the TENS and its use, stop the treatment. These problems can usually be resolved at your next review. If your next review is more than a week away, contact the clinic through one of the numbers at the end of the booklet.

HOW LONG CAN I KEEP THE TENS FOR?

The trial usually takes around six weeks. During this time, you will be seen up to five times when the machines may be adjusted and the electrodes moved to get the best pain control for you. At the end of this period, it is your responsibility to return the TENS machine on your last review.

WHERE DO I GET A MACHINE FOR LONGER USE?

If you have had a good result with TENS, you may consider purchasing your own machine. Ask the advice of your clinician before you buy a machine as there are some for sale which do not offer all the facilities that you may need.

DO...

- Use your TENS daily as directed by your clinician. (You will receive lots of advice from other people but please stick to the directions that you have been given by your pain clinic).

- Keep your skin clean and inspect where the electrodes go daily. If you have any skin problems, stop using the TENS until your next visit to the clinic.

- Take care of your machine.

- Place the electrodes on the plastic film overnight.

- Keep your appointments. You may have up to five reviews when the internal controls of the TENS may be adjusted to achieve the best pain management for you.

DON'T...

- Don't loan the machine to anyone else.

- Don't get the machine wet.

- Don't stick the electrodes together.

- Don't kink the wires or pull the plugs out of the machine by the wires.

KINGS Professionals' Guide to TENS

Electrode Positions

The provision of a body plan allows the clinician to illustrate electrode positions.

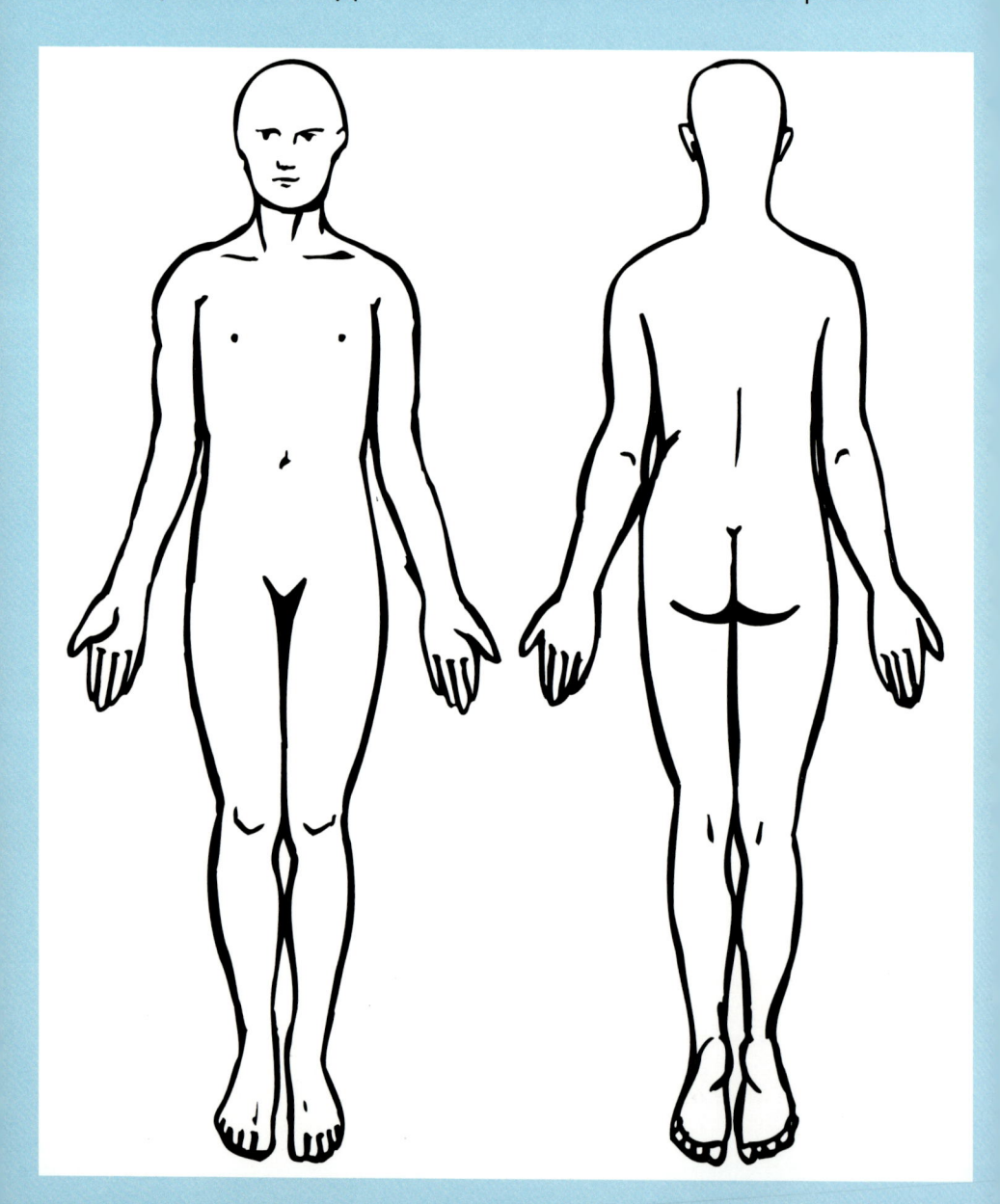

KINGS Professionals' Guide to TENS

Clinicians Name:

Telephone Number:

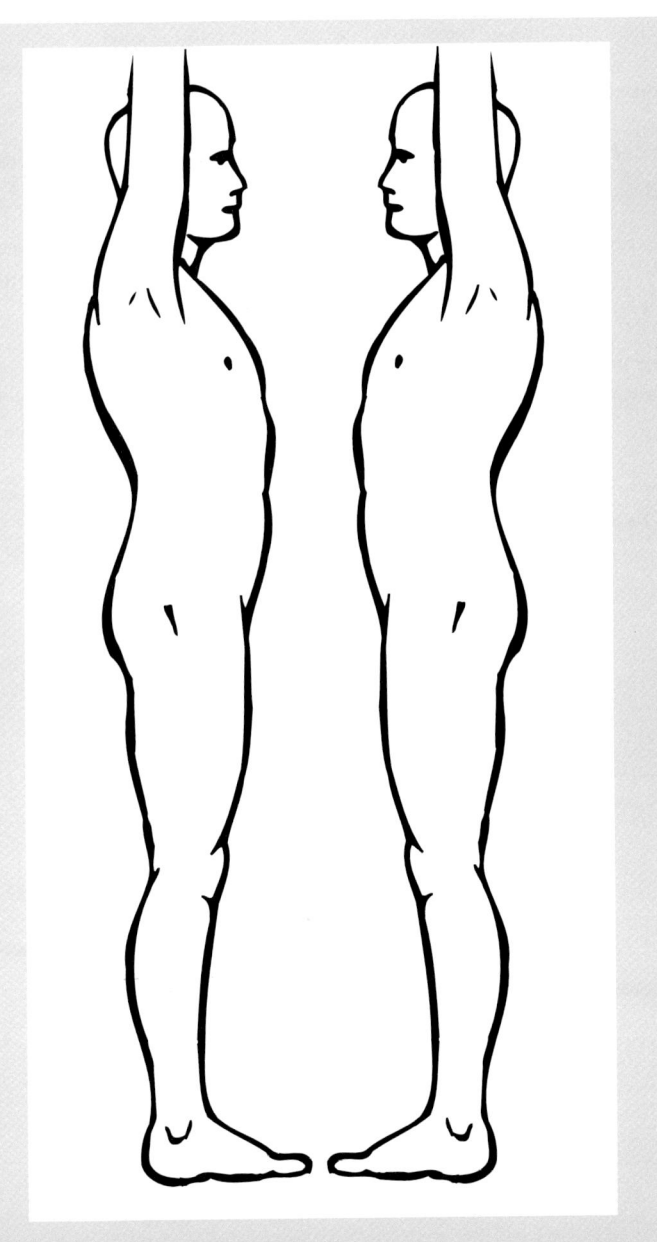

Conclusion

The most important first step in a trial of TENS with a patient is the time spent in explaining that the most likely outcome of treatment may be a reduction in pain or achieving pain management rather than a cure! It is also important at this time to stress that it may take several visits and adjustments before any benefit may be perceived.

The importance of a full assessment and the recording of present linear pain scales, sleep patterns and levels of function cannot be over emphasised.

Your may find it necessary to "fine tune" electrode positions as each major nerve has contributions form several nerve roots. Happily, these are adjacent vertebrae therefore moving the centrally placed electrode up or down one segment may suffice.

If, after following the guide to "anatomical" electrode placement, you have not achieved significant pain management, Acupuncture points offer an electrical window on the nervous system.

Treating pain with TENS is not a cure all. However, if the clinician follows a logical progression of treatment, the most significant results may be achieved

Alan King

References

1. Melzack R, Wall P D. Pain Mechanisms: a New Theory. Science. 1965; 150: 971-979
2. Eriksson M B E, Sjölund B H, Nielzen S. Long Term Results of Peripheral Conditioning Stimulation as an Analgesic Measure in Chronic Pain. Pain. 1979; 6: 335-347.
3. Walsh D M. TENS Clinical Applications and Related Theory. 1997; Churchill Livingstone.

    ISBN 0-443-05323-5
4. Han J, Wang Q. Mobilization of Specific Neuropeptides by Peripheral Stimulation of Identified Frequencies. News in Physiological Sciences. 1992; 7. 176-180.
5. Merskey H, Albe-Fassard D G, Bronica J J et al. Pain terms: A list with definitions and notes on usage. Pain. 1979; 6: 249-252.
6. Oden R V, Postoperative Pain; Incidence and Severity in; Ferrante Ostheimer Corino (eds).

    Oxford: Blackwell. 1990 10-6
7. Tachi N et al, Muscle involvement in congenital insensitivity to pain with anhidrosis. Pediatric Neurology. 1995; 12 (3) 264-266.
8. Rosemberg S, Marie S K, Klienman S. Congenital insensitivity to pain with Anhidrosis.

    Paediatric Neurology. 1994; 11 (1): 50-6.
9. Hirsch E, Moye D, Dimon J H. Congenital indifference to pain.

    Southern Medical Journal. 1995; 88 (8): 851-857.
10. Barr M L, Kiernan. The Human Nervous System. Fourth Edition.

    Published by Harper and Row. 1983. ISBN 0-06-140311-3
11. Campbell J N, Taub A. Local Analgesia from Percutaneous Electrical Stimulation. A peripheral Mechanism. Arch. Neurol (Chic), 1973. 28. 347-350.
12. Garrison D W, Foreman D F. Decreased activity of spontaneous and noxiously evoked dorsal horn cells during transcutaneous electrical nerve stimulation (TENS). Pain. 1994; 58: 309-315.
13. Wang S F, Chen Y W, Shyu B C. The suppressive effect of electrical stimulation on nociceptive responses in the rat. Physical Therapy. 1997; 77 (8) 839-847.
14. Salar G, Job I, Mingrino S, Bosio A, Trabucchi M. Effect of Transcutaneous Electrotherapy on CSF Beta-Endorphin Content in Patients Without Pain Problems. Pain. 1981; 10. 169-172.
15. Sjölund B H, Eriksson M B E. The Influence on Analgesia Produced by Peripheral Conditioning Stimulation. Brain Research. 1979; 173. 295-301.
16. Green J H. An Introduction to Human Physiology. Fourth S.I. Ed. Oxford Medical Publications. 1985. ISBN 0-19-263328-7.
17. Gyton A C. Textbook of Medical Physiology. Seventh Ed. W.B. Saunders Company. 1986. ISBN 0-7216-1260-1.

18. Williams P L, Warwick R. Ed's. Gray's Anatomy. 36th Edition. Churchill Livingstone. 1984. ISBN 0-443-01505-8.

19. Wells P E, Framton V, Bowsher D. Pain Management by Physiotherapy. Second Ed. Butterworth Heinman 1994. 54-58. ISBN 0-7506-3084-1.

20. Charman R A. Pain Theory and Physiotherapy. Physiotherapy. 1989; 75 (5). 247-54.

21. Igneizi R J, Nyquist J K. Direct Effect of Electrical Stimulation on Peripheral Nerve Evoked Activity: Implications on Pain Relief. Journal of Neurosurgery. 1976; 45. 159-165.

22. Igneizi R J, Nyquist J K. Excitability Changes in Peripheral Nerves after Repetitive Electrical Stimulation: Implications in Pain Modulation. Journal of Neurosurgery. 1979; 51. 824-833.

23. Sjölund B H, Eriksson M B E. Endorphins and Analgesia Produced by Peripheral Conditioning Stimulation. Advances in Pain Research and Therapy. 1979; Vol. 3, edited by John J Bronica et al. Raven Press, New York.

24. Melzack R, Wall P. The Challenge of Pain. New Edition. 1988; Penguin Books. ISBN 0-14-022709-1.

25. Sjölund B, Eriksson M. Relief of Pain by TENS. 1985. John Wiley and Sons. IBSN 0-471-90753-7.

26. Johnson M I, Aston C H, Bousfield D R, Thompson J W. Analgesic effects of Different Pulse Patterns of Transcutaneous Electrical Nerve Stimulation on Cold Induced Pain in Normal Subjects. Journal of Psychosomatic Research. 1991 Vol. 35; 2/3. 313-321.

27. Sjölund B, Eriksson M. Electro-Acupuncture and Endogenous Morphines. Lancet. November 1976.1085.

28. Sjölund B, Eriksson M. The Influence of Naloxone on Analgesia Produced by Peripheral Conditioning Stimulation. Brain Research. 1979; 173. 295-301.

29. Eriksson M, Sjölund B. Acupuncture Like Electroanalgesia in TNS Resistant Chronic Pain. Chapter in Sensory Functions of The Skin.1976. Ed Y Zoterman. Pergamon Press, Oxford. 575-581.

30. Librach S L, Rapson L M. The Use of Transcutaneous Electrical Nerve Stimulation (TENS) for the relief of pain in palliative Care. Palliative Medicine.1988; 2. 15-20.

31. Sjölund B H, Eriksson M, Loeser J D. Transcutaneous and Implanted Electrical Stimulation of Peripheral Nerves. Management of Pain. 2nd edition: 1990. John Bonica. Lea and Febiger. 1852-1861.

32. Mannheimer J S. Electrode Placements for Transcutaneous Electrical Nerve Stimulation. Physical Therapy. 1978; 58 (12). 1455-1462.

33. Casey K L, Blick M. Observations on Anodal Polarisation of Cutaneous Nerve. Brain Research. 1969; 13. 155-167.

34. Mendell L M, Wall P D. Presynaptic Hyperpolarisation: A role for Fine Afferent Fibres. Journal of Physiology. 1964; 172. 274-294.

35. Lockhart R D, Hamilton G F, Fyfe F W. Anatomy of the Human Body. Faber. 1965. ISBN 0-571-0703J-X

36. McMinn R M H, Hutchings R T, Pegington J, Abrahams P. A Colour Atlas of Human Anatomy. Third Edition. Mosby-Wolfe. 1995. ISBN 0-7234-1915-9.

37. Berlant S R. Method of Determining Optimal Stimulation Sites for Transcutaneous Electrical Nerve Stimulation. Physical Therapy. 1984; 64 (6). 924-928.
38. Wolf S L, Gersh M R, Rao V R. Examination of Electrode Placements and Stimulating Parameters in Treating Chronic Pain With Conventional Transcutaneous Electrical Nerve Stimulation (TENS).

    Pain. 1981; 11. 37-47.
39. Szeto A Y J, Nyquist J K. Transcutaneous Electrical Nerve Stimulation for Pain Control. IEEE Engineering in Medicine and Biology Magazine. Dec' 1983. 14-26.
40. Han J S, Chen X H, Sun S L, Xu X J, Yuan Y, Yan S C, Hao J X, Terenius L. Effect of low- and high frequency TENS on Met-enkephalin-Arg-Phe and dynorphin A immunoreactivity in human lumbar CSF. Pain. 1991; 47. 295-298.
41. Lundeberg T. Electrical Stimulation for the Relief of Pain. Physiotherapy. 1984; 70 (3). 98-100.
42. Marshall P. TENS in chronic angina. Professional Nurse. October 1991; 20-22.
43. Grimmer K. A controlled double blind study comparing the effects of strong burst mode TENS and high rate TENS on painful osteoarthritic knees. Australian Physiotherapy. 1992; 38 (1). 49-56.
44. Reading A E. The McGill Pain Questionnaire: an appraisal; in R Melzack (ed) Pain Measurement and Assessment. Raven Press, New York, 1983 55-61.
45. Marchand S, Li J, Charest J. Effects of Caffeine on Analgesia from Transcutaneous Electrical Nerve Stimulation. The New England Journal of Medicine. Aug' 1995; 333. 325-326.
46. Dundee J W, Ghaly R G, Bill K M, Chestnutt W N, Fitzpatrick K T J, Lynas A G A. Effect of Stimulation of the P6 Antiemetic Point on Postoperative Nausea and Vomiting.

    British Journal of Anaesthesia. 1989; 63. 612-618.
47. Al-Sadi M, Newman B, Julious S A. Acupuncture in the Prevention of Postoperative Nausea and Vomiting. Anaesthesia. 1997; 52. 658-661.
48. McMillan C M, Dundee J W. The Role of Transcutaneous Electrical Nerve Stimulation of Neiguan Anti-Emetic Acupuncture Point in Controlling Sickness After Cancer Chemotherapy.

    Physiotherapy. 1991; 77, (7). 449-502.

Index

A-beta nerves - 15, **17**
Action potential - 14
Acupuncture-like TENS - 28
Acute pain - 13
A-delta nerves - 15, **18**
Afferent pathways - 15
Allergies - 47
Amplitude - 48
Anti-emisis - 46
Arthritis - 14
Assessment - 40

Biphasic pulse - 23
Burst stimulation - 25-26, 48

Caffeine (effects on TENS) - 47
Cautions to using TENS - 12
Central nervous system - 15, 20
Cervical spine - 34
C fibres - 18
Chemotherapy - 46
Chronic pain - 13
Circulation 6 - 46
CNS (see Central nervous system)
Collaterals - 18
Constant stimulation - 24, 48
Contact allergies - 47
Contra-indications - 12

Depolorisation - 14
Dermatomal stimulation - 31
Dermatome - 32, *34-35*,
Dorsal Column Stimulation - 8
Duration of treatment - 36

Electrical burn - 47
ELECTRODE
    Allergy to - 47
    Choosing the right ones - 49
    Polarity - 30-32
    Positioning - 32-33
    Sites - 33
Endogenous opioids - 12, 18, 21, 24, 26, **28-29, 37**

First order neurones - 15, **17**,
Frequency of treatment - 36
Frequently asked questions - 50-53

Headaches - 47
Hyperpolarisation - 31-32
Hypotension - 47

Indications for treatment - 38
Injury without pain - 13
Interneurones - 15

Keeping notes - 40

Lead wires - 49
Locating vertebrae - 34
Lumbar spine - 34
Lymphoedema - 47

McGill pain questionnaire - 40
Mobility - 11
Modality - 48
Monophasic waveform - 24
Myelin sheath - 17
Myotome - 32

Naloxone - 21
Nausea - 46
Negative electrode - 30-32
NERVES
    Introduction - 14
    Of the CNS - 20
    Peripheral - 17, 19
Neuropathic pain - 38
Nociceptive pain - 38
Nociceptor - 18
Non steroidal anti-inflammatories - 11
Normal stimulation - 24
Notes - 40
NSAI - 11

Opioids (see Endogenous Opioids)
Osteo-arthritis - 14

Pacinian corpuscles - 15
PAIN
    Acute - 13
    Chronic - 13
    Definitions of - 13
    Pain without injury - 14
Pain-gate - 12, 17, 19, 21, 24, 26, **37**,
Pain management programme - 38
Periaqueductal grey matter - 21
Peripheral nerves - 17
Peripheral neuropathies - 37
Polarity of electrodes - 30
Positive electrode - 30-32
Positioning the electrodes - 32-33
Pregnancy - 46, 50
Proprioception - 17
Psychiatric evaluation - 39
Psychological overlay - 39
Pulse duration - 48

References - 56, 57
Refractory period - 14
Reviews of progress - 40-41
Rheumatoid arthritis - 14

Second order neurones - 15, 20
Side effects to using TENS - 47
Single bi-phasic pulse - 23
Substantia Gelatinosa - 8, 18, 19

TENS
    Advantages of - 10-11
    Cautions and Contra-indications - 12
    Choosing equipment - 48
    Do's and Don'ts - 53
    Genesis of - 8
    Introduction to - 7
    Machine - 22, 48
    Neuromodulation of pain - 21
    Output - 23
    Overview of - 12
    Setting the machine - 26
    Side-effects - 47
Thalamic pain - 16
Third order neurones - 20
Thoracic spine - 34
TREATMENT
    Duration - 36
    Indications - 38

Vertebrae - how to locate them - 34

Wind-up phenomenon - 47

ADDITIONAL NOTES

ADDITIONAL NOTES

ADDITIONAL NOTES